I FLY OUT
WITH BRIGHT FEATHERS

ALLEGRA TAYLOR was born in 1940 and had an uncon-
ventional, globe-trotting childhood with no formal
education. At seventeen, she married film-maker Richard
Taylor and they now have five grown-up children, two of
whom they adopted while living in Nigeria. While the
children were young, she took a degree in Music and
Education and spent many years teaching music in her
local community. She is also a freelance journalist and
has written a children's book about life on a kibbutz.

ALLEGRA TAYLOR

I FLY OUT
WITH BRIGHT
FEATHERS

The Quest of a Novice Healer

SAFFRON WALDEN
THE C. W. DANIEL COMPANY LIMITED

First published in 1987 by William Collins, London

This edition was first published in 1992 by
The C.W. Daniel Company Limited
1 Church Path, Saffron Walden, Essex CB10 1JP, England

ISBN 0 85207 267 8

Produced by Ennisfield Print & Design
Wapping, London

For my parents Pat and Camille
who taught me that love is possible.

ACKNOWLEDGEMENTS

Many people have helped and encouraged me in the writing of this book. In particular I would like to thank:

All the healers I met who so generously gave of their knowledge and wisdom; Kenya Airways, for their generosity in sponsoring my trip to Kenya; Toby Eady, my literary agent, for believing in me; Carol O'Brien and Simon King of Collins for taking the gamble; Amanda Langford for her valuable comments and hard work on the manuscript; Georgina Guttridge, my great friend, for her tremendous labour of typing it all onto a word processor; my beloved children for not letting me take myself too seriously; and, above all, Richard my husband for his constant love and support.

I

I Fly Out With Bright Feathers

The day my mother died and I sat for a while beside her poor old body, I took her hands in mine — now as fragile as ancient parchment — and remembered as if it were yesterday the feel of her gentle, loving touch bringing me comfort and healing when I was ill as a child. Enfolding me in a certainty of belonging. Acceptance without judgement, the sweetest sensation in the world.

We instinctively put our arms around a frightened child, an injured friend, a grief-stricken neighbour — holding a hand in sympathy, soothing a troubled brow or stroking a feverish cheek. Healing, as I understand it, is an extension of that instinct — of something we all, in our more sensitive moments, use naturally.

I was moved by a tentative altruistic notion to want to help and heal others, to be able to offer something more useful than just a sympathetic ear to friends in time of sorrow or pain. Something practical.

'Pardon me, but I think my karma has just run over your dogma,' a voice boomed in my ear as I milled with the crowds at the Festival for Mind and Body at Olympia. A medieval soothsayer introduced himself as Melchior. He was dressed in tattered sacking and bindings like a film extra from a King Arthur movie and carried on a little dialogue with his wayward walking stick as we chatted. 'It tends to get a bit restless when it's indoors,' he explained, but eventually managed to calm it down by taking the rubber stopper off the end.

He embodied everything both hilarious and off-putting about

the alternative lifestyle and spiritual growth movement that had always prevented me from taking it seriously or attempting a closer acquaintance. But on this occasion I had overcome my own considerable resistance and gone along to see what I could see. I was met by a bewildering array of services on offer; from goat's milk to gurus, from fairground charlatans praising the properties of magic crystals to earnest representatives of alternative farming communities wearing organic sandals – each one guaranteeing improved health and/or spiritual enlightenment. I thought I could feel some healing ability in my hands and I was looking for an affirmation that my first timid efforts were gropings in the right direction.

I had also once had a strange experience that opened, in my mind, a door to a much bigger room. It hadn't exactly frightened me but it left me in awe of its strength and power. My youngest son had been having a lot of difficulties in his life. He was sickly, skinny and unhappy at school and I didn't know how to help him. One night I was stroking his hair as he slept fitfully and feeling a great accumulation of helplessness. I suddenly had an irresistible impulse to raise my hand above my head. I am not a religious believer but I thrust it upwards rather self-consciously, glad no one was watching me, in a gesture of great yearning and desperation. Almost immediately, my whole arm began to tingle as if I'd come into contact with a stream of effervescent energy particles. His little body became calm and peaceful and I had a sense of mighty, surging power surrounding us. I knew then, with absolute certainty, that something stronger than me, something collective, was there when I needed to draw on it. It occurred to me that perhaps a healer can operate from an *intention* which utilizes the natural harmonious energy of the universe. Could I learn to harness this energy? Could I use it to be a better mother, a better friend? Human beings seem to be connected to each other in some mysterious way. Perhaps a person's broken-down immune system can be sparked off again by another person's energy like the jump leads on a car battery. Can the mind play a part – reversing the disease process by an act of will or faith? After all, if fear, hate and jealousy can produce profound chemical changes in the body, why not love? How do miracle cures happen? We need each other, we need help. Could the laying on of hands be seen as a sort of nourishment?

I am certainly not alone in recognizing that we are each a unique combination of mind, body and spirit that should be working in harmonious balance to produce well-being – rather than a collection of spare parts to be serviced. And although Western scientific medicine has achieved a remarkable level of technological brilliance, it also has its limitations. It has not proved very effective in dealing with diseases such as cancer and arthritis, for example, and people are becoming alarmed about the addictive properties and side-effects of certain drugs which can prove more horrific than the disease they were meant to eradicate in the first place.

Brian Inglis, in his book *Fringe Medicine*, puts it well: 'Why should we reject the possibility of healing forces when it is easier to believe that they exist than that all the evidence for them has been due to a combination of error, misunderstanding, coincidence, gullibility and fraud perpetrated by the unscrupulous on the credulous or by the credulous on each other?'

In spite of the hostility and suspicion shown towards healing by the medical profession, over a million people a year consult healers in Britain and the Church is beginning to revive its healing ministry. What attracts me so much to this type of healing is its simplicity and the fact that it can't do any harm. It is not a complicated system of diagnoses and remedies but seems to work on the level of unselfish love and compassion. Not an emotional love which is bound up with one's own needs, but a caring, unconditional, detached love with no beginning and no end. It should be complementary to other forms of healing and medical practice and not in any kind of conflict with them.

My first tentative steps on the healing trail began at that festival of esoterica as I browsed among the stalls selling embossed plastic runes (including instructions) for amateur sages, magic wands and crystal balls, De Luxe Pyramid Energy Kits with which to sharpen your razor blades and bottles of jinx-removing oil.

When I saw Andrew Watson's Five-Day Healing Intensive

advertised as 'Self-Healing and Energy Balancing' I wasn't sure it was quite the right thing for me. Self-healing? There was nothing the matter with me, but I went to hear him speak and he seemed to have a lot of good things to say and a likable, direct manner so right there and then I signed on for the course.

A young Nigerian friend talking about passing his school exams once said to me in a delightful adaptation of 'coming through with flying colours': 'I fly out with bright feathers.' I think that rather suits me. Cheerful, noisy and an easy target – trespassing presumptuously where only theologians and philosophers usually dare to tread. This is really the story of my own idiosyncratic journey of discovery. It's not an academic thesis or an encyclopaedia of techniques, but a personal search for an understanding of the healing phenomenon.

I was looking forward to the course a lot but my obvious anxiety and tension on the first day took me by surprise. I overslept and arrived late with a sty in my eye and a headache indicating more mixed feelings than I cared to recognize. There were about eighteen people, all ages, more women than men, and the course was held in a large airy upstairs room full of cushions and sofas in a private house.

Andrew began by playing a tape of monotonous meditation-type music to get us in the right mood. A bad start – I found it irritating, very self-conscious and moony. My heart sank a bit and I could feel the sensible British side of my nature beginning to defend itself against infiltration. But then Jules, his co-leader, read a Sufi fable about a stream trying to cross a desert. Time and time again it soaks into the sand, and only once it realizes that it must give up its vapour to the sun and allow itself to be transformed into a cloud is it able at last to be transported. I took the hint. Okay, I'll keep an open mind.

Andrew then demonstrated some astonishing evidence of the power of the mind using mental images of energy flowing through the body, creating invincible strength. This is the resource used by some forms of oriental martial arts such as aikido and, although Andrew was using a party trick format for the purposes of the demonstration, seeing something before my very eyes was a good way to convince me.

He stood in the middle of the room with one arm outstretched to the side and invited someone to come forward and bend it. it was easily done, of course, as the arm in that position, unbraced, has very little strength. Then, with his arm in the same position, he said he was visualizing it as a fire hose turned full on with water roaring through it at high pressure. 'Now nothing on earth can bend it,' he said, and invited the strongest person in the room to try. He was perfectly relaxed and apparently using no muscular force but no one could bend the fire hose. Then he did a similar demonstration forming a circle with the index finger and thumb of one hand; easily broken until he visualized an iron ring. We all tried it ourselves and found, with great excitement, that it worked. Even as beginners we could start using and conveying the power of this energy flow. We worked in pairs, massaging each other to feel what it is like both to give and receive. Glimmers. Jules read another Sufi fable about a group of blind men all thinking they understand what an elephant is because they have each touched a different part, but all their definitions are different and none of them has grasped the whole picture.

We faced each other with eyes closed, lightly touching palms, trying in turn to transmit and receive 'unconditional love' from the heart chakra. I didn't as yet understand about chakras but my heart felt full. Definite stirrings. The first real evidence for me that intention is picked up by the receiver. After the lunch break we tried a directed drawing exercise. You have to imagine yourself first as a tree, then an animal, a bird, an insect and a part of the earth, and draw them on different sheets of paper. The idea is to empty your mind and try to trust the first idea or image that occurs to you as it can quite often give you some surprising insight into the state of your unconscious. My tree was a flourishing one. Many branches, new young leaves in springtime, strong deep roots nearly as plentiful as the part above ground. A safe nesting place for a bird. My animal was a surprise to me, quite a shock in fact; I saw a large moose with a very mournful expression and enormous antlers weighing down his head. He was standing knee-deep in a lake and there was a faceless hunter behind a bush aiming a gun at him. The whole image was suffused with a feeling of unbearable sadness and doom. My bird drawing was of a huge black condor soaring above sharp-pointed, snow-capped, inhospitable-looking mountain peaks, trying in vain to find a place to land but warmed by a vibrant life-giving sun in the sky. It spoke to me simultaneously of loneliness and liberty. My insect was a busy jolly fat green caterpillar walking along a stem towards green leaves – on a journey of physical and spiritual fulfilment? On its way to metamorphosis? And my part of the earth was a pale desert of shifting sands defined by a distant horizon and guided by a lone star.

They all seemed interesting, relevant to me and curiously linked to one another. Only the moose bothered me. Why the resignation? Why the doom? Were the antlers a symbol of something I wanted to shed? A responsibility that weighed me down? A trophy for the unseen hunter? Had I allowed myself to be a victim like so many women: exposed, vulnerable, pathetic, helpless? Were my recurring headaches the antlers, the metaphorical 'weight on my mind'? The image was mine. I made it. I would have to own it and take responsibility for it. I would have to face it and come to terms with it. What truth had I stumbled upon? Andrew said I should contact the image in a guided meditation, try to communicate with it, ask the animal what it was saying to me.

This is very akin to North American Indian practice where animal guides are very powerful figures and come in dreams and states of heightened awareness with vital messages for those with ears to hear. I would have to listen to my moose.

Our next exercise was to form ourselves into groups of three and attempt some amateur interpretation of each other's drawings. My tragic moose was a Jewish racial memory, suggested my friend Ruth who had also come on the course. Maybe. Her drawings were interesting in the light of her frail ego and proclivity for cataclysmic depressions – a stick-like, unformed tree, a bat, a newly hatched chick, a radiant butterfly, and an exploding volcano.

We paired again and experimented with different partners, trying to send energy first to the right then to the left, seeing if the partner could sense the direction. Very strong response. I could feel a lot of power in my left hand and visualized the energy as a core of golden particles washing through my arms like sea waves. Andrew suggested that before going to sleep that night we should ask for a clear and easily remembered dream. A good habit to get into is to write your dreams down. We finished that first astonishing, thought-provoking day by linking into a circle with our arms around each other and creating a projection of love energy going first one way round then the other and finally into a pool from which we could each drink our fill and satisfy our thirst. Twenty-four hours before, I might have found it all a bit toe-curling but now our little group, who were all strangers that morning, seemed like travelling companions setting off on a sea voyage with nothing to be gained by keeping one foot on the quayside. I hoped I was sufficiently aware of the Emperor's New Clothes syndrome not to fall victim to the dangers of longing to belong. I knew I would just have to trust my common sense, my relative sanity, and my sense of humour to help me preserve my critical faculties at the same time as I vaporized to cross the desert.

I awoke the next morning sweating with fright, heart thumping from a graphic, vivid dream, terribly real, that my second son, Tim, had died. I had come home and found him slumped on the stairs with the other children clustered round in anxiety. He'd just fallen there, dead of a brain haemorrhage. I held him and wept and wept until my chest hurt. I found a postcard he had written and I read it out to my husband. It was pitifully illiterate and brave. 'Don't miss me I have to go home,' it said. I felt guilty that I hadn't been a good enough mother to him, that I had failed him where I hadn't failed the others. My head throbbed and I felt deeply upset and disturbed by the dream. This was going to be a more painful journey than I'd thought.

Andrew led us in a deeper process of discovery about the meaning of our images, a guided meditation. We each chose something from yesterday to focus on, closed our eyes and imagined leaving our known selves above the ground and journeying deep down into the earth. I decided to enter wholeheartedly into the spirit of this and not resist it just because it was unfamiliar and had echoes of joke séances about it. Visualization, the creation of mind pictures, is a central and recurring concept in healing work. It can play an important role in revealing old patterns of response and preparing the mind for the desired changes. I descended an infinite ladder, seeing above me a diminishing speck of light, very small and weak, as I went further and further into the depths of the unknown. I came at last to a ledge where I could rest, where secrets would be revealed, and where images could speak to me. I learnt instantly that the person holding the gun in my picture was myself. My own worst enemy? The poor resigned moose had no need to stand there bogged down and passive. The antlers could be shed. I still wasn't sure what the antlers represented. Indecision? Clutter? A lot of clutter in my life. Very thin ankles in the water. Stuck in the mud and easily snapped if I try to run away. It might be easier to move on without all that heavy weight on my head.

We all found that it was possible to have a dialogue with the subconscious mind in this semi-trance state and masses of useful insights came into focus. My dear worried friend Ruth was visited by just about the whole gamut of mythological archetypes during her journey to the centre of the earth: sword, chalice, scarab, pyramid, star of David.

Jules is excellent at Jungian dream analysis and interpretation and very knowledgeable about the legends and fairy stories in which these ancient symbols occur all over the world. I have heard doctors and counsellors complain that stirring up these seething cauldrons is dangerous and irresponsible, leaving people vulnerable and exposed – their cover blown. Certainly anyone dabbling should be aware of the power of such analysis. I see it as a valuable tool to be used with care. After all, a sharp knife is indispensable in the kitchen, a motor car a boon on a long journey, but in the hands of a maniac or a potential suicide either could be lethal. I suppose the secret once again is to know in your own mind when you are ready to ask questions of yourself and assume responsibility for the answers, no matter how unlikely these turn out to be.

Our group had begun to create its own special dynamic – a fascinating phenomenon to watch in action. As human beings we seem to want to create a little tribe wherever there exist likely components, shared interests, similar goals and a few small ceremonies or rituals to act as a binding agent (like church hymns, club rules, secret signs, rugby songs). In this group we had no option but to trust each other or the whole thing would be a flop. We all wanted and needed to trust each other – everyone there was seeking a sanctuary where it would be safe to turn inside out, where no one would ridicule you or take advantage of you with your guard down. There are very few places in our competitive, survival-of-the-fittest society where we can relax our constant watchfulness and share our secrets.

One exercise we did this morning was to explore each other's hands. We sat facing each other with our eyes closed and felt our own hands, then explored each other's for a long time. Curious to be so intimate with a stranger, but because our intentions towards each other weren't in the least erotic, there were only very faint sexual connotations; mainly a strong awareness of each trying to give the other what he or she most needed. It was quite a long exercise and changed in character from being playful, to still, to healing back and forth. My partner felt quite moved by the end of it and a bit tearful. I felt conscious of having absorbed something of her into myself in a strange sort of way – an essence which enabled me to understand her without words. I was also struck by the fact that all this is so easy once one is given the permission to do it. Pathetic how one needs this affirmation to feel at ease doing something that should be so normal and natural. Why not do it more often in other situations?

Later we talked about our dreams and I found it almost unbearably painful to recount mine. My breath got short and my chest tight. Many of us had experienced troubled dreams that

17

night so the next thing we tried was a lengthy healing body massage on a different partner, stopping halfway to discuss how it felt.

We learned the Golden Waterfall Meditation. You imagine yourself soaring on a magic carpet, flying high, floating in the scented air until you come upon an immense golden waterfall pouring through space, through infinity, showering you with particles of radiant golden light. You drift silently through it while the light funnels in through the top of your head and down your arms to the person on the receiving end. This was very effective and I found it easy to do. I felt a strong tingling sensation of healing energy coming out of my left hand which had the somewhat disconcerting effect of making my partner very weepy. The idea was to trust your intuition so I just held her feet gently and firmly and tried to send her a calming warmth. There were suddenly a lot of tears in the room, a lot of pent-up feelings, but everyone responded to the loving touch treatment. The massage I received was an interesting experience, positively pulsating. Intuition led my partner to place her hands on my joints — shoulders, knees, elbows, ankles and wrists and to connect them up with a gentle transmission of energy. I got a lot of soothing heat from her hands and felt very refreshed afterwards. We all shared the good we'd brought and talked like old friends. For the last exercise of the day I worked with Ted, a vet, who had used healing on his animals with quite a lot of success. He was a very gentle man who felt himself ineffectual in a hostile world; his dreams were of planes that wouldn't fly. This was a hand-touching thing again, transmitting and receiving a current of energy. The point of the exercise this time was to resist our partner's flow as hard as possible and they had to try any devious means to sneak the energy in. I found it absolutely exhausting to resist; my whole arm ached with the effort as if I was trying to hold back a wall that was crushing me. Then, when we could permit the flow again, it rushed through like pumping blood when a tourniquet is removed, and we could both feel the reciprocal transmission very strongly. We finished by spending some time with each other's most blocked and tense area of the body. Mine was my neck and shoulders, his was the heart area of his chest. It was good to surrender the tension in such an atmosphere of mutual trust. My lingering headache lifted at last. We all stood a few moments at the end of the day with our arms around each other feeling vitalized and rested.

I had hoped for a dream of some significance that night but I had none that I could remember; all night long, however, and still as I awoke in the morning, my arms were aching from the resistance-to-energy exercise. Real muscular stiffness, as if I'd been doing weight-lifting, but of course it was all in my mind. It made me realize how much energy we expend in our everyday lives doing nothing but defending ourselves against other people, and underlined again how physical all this mental stuff is.

First partner exercise today was with Christopher, a man so pathologically shy and self-effacing as to be almost invisible. We began with transmitting through the hands, then tried to send a beam of energy from one heart to the other. We were meant to try and open our hearts to receive an image or intuition about the person we were with. I felt Christopher to be a man with a lot of love to give but very little self-confidence, especially with women − such timid energy came from him, like Tinkerbell's fading light after drinking the poison in *Peter Pan*. We attempted to transmit through the eyes, opening them and staring deep into the windows of the soul. This is a very intimate thing to do and it requires a great deal of trust. Normally only lovers or mothers and babies gaze at each other in this way. It was the first time we'd done anything with our eyes open and I felt very uneasy about my own being looked into so searchingly to begin with. I wasn't at all sure I wanted to be so exposed, so transparent. But I soon got so involved with his eyes that I stopped worrying. After a short while his face began to distort. I saw a whole row of eyes going round his head and then a face with no eyes at all, symbolizing to me alternate states of watchfulness and hiding. When I shared with him my rather presumptuous intuitive feelings about his character, he was astonished that I'd guessed so much. It occurred to me that perhaps psychics, palmists and clairvoyants work on this level − using the tarot or tea-leaves or

19

whatever as a springboard, but basically getting information from their highly tuned intuitive faculties. Christopher was very upset because he felt nothing and said he couldn't visualize anything. In fact I felt quite a lot coming from him. He gives more than he knows and it was pitiful to see how little self-esteem he had.

The next long process I did was with an elderly widower of abundant charm and old-world courtesy. A healing again, trying to use the intuitions gained from touch to focus on the person's needy areas. Again I felt slight tensions and conflicts surrendering to a man especially since the one being treated was supposed actively to assist by being as receptive and as yielding as they could. In fact I found the dear old man most tender and safe, very caring and gentle like an ideal father. It was altogether a lovely experience, an infant pleasure. Learning to trust is as important as learning to give.

Later we did what is called a sub-personality exercise where you float off into a guided meditation and try to visualize a house full of rooms with closed doors. You are supposed to enter the house, open all the doors and confront the people behind them – all different aspects of yourself. The idea is to speak to them and invite them outside into a meadow, in order to recognize and try to integrate the various facets of your personality. I pictured a Wild West Saloon with a balcony and sort of brothel-type rooms leading off. I opened and shut the doors quickly. I didn't like what I saw. In the first room was a little girl with pigtails and wet knickers – I knew it was me at five years old, embarrassed and ashamed. Next door was a spotty-faced teenage girl with an ugly, unbecoming haircut, unpopular and awkward: me at thirteen. In the next room was a large white polar bear, male, that tried to escape but I shut him in again, and finally, in the last room, an evil goat-like figure with wiry limbs and luminous yellow eyes hiding behind the large jolly figure of a baker in white floury clothes who filled the doorway and blocked it. Maybe I wasn't quite ready to face the nastier aspects of my personality? Afterwards we discussed these experiences in small groups. Poor Christopher had terrible creatures behind his doors and he began to sob as if it was the end of the world. The girl near him held him in her arms and he cried and cried. I felt very distressed by his pain although glad for him that he could express it. He looked much better afterwards and everyone gave him lots of love. The atmosphere of the group with its shared common purpose was extraordinarily supportive.

The last exercise of the day was a threesome meditation. We tried to construct in our midst an imaginary triangle filled with a pyramid of energy. It was magically successful for all of us, and the first time I had not been bothered by intrusive trivialities in my meditation. This was pure light that just lifted me away. We all held each other again in a circle of love and acceptance feeling very close and homogeneous, hardly wanting to break apart.

I was aware that night of many dreams going on but they vanished with the morning. I felt wonderful, very invigorated and potent. At the beginning of that day people shared their dreams, then we paired off for a partner exercise. The idea was to sit facing but not quite touching and look deeply into one another's eyes. The difference from previous exercises was the absence of physical contact. With eyes alone what was it possible to learn about your partner and about yourself?

While I was doing this exercise I had no idea if what I was seeing was a projection of my imagination or if it was really happening, but I went along with it anyway, riding my perceptions as though white-water rafting. First we were asked to focus on each other's left eye and I began to feel an overwhelming sadness. I saw pain and vulnerability. I was overtaken by a sense of identification and common genetic inheritance. I started to become her! I could see more of my father and myself in her face than I could of her. Both of us had tears trickling down. Very odd. But the strangest part was how different gazing into the right eye was. I could glare at her coldly, I didn't blink and no tears came. The eye staring back at me was judgemental and unforgiving and again I realized I was seeing myself. We had to focus on the area of the third eye, the so-called 'brow chakra', and try to pierce through and beyond, letting the face blur. I couldn't see anything but laughter, forgiveness and carefreeness.

Oh well, I thought, vivid imagination, very suggestible; but then we started discussing our perceptions. My partner had also felt the same sadness on the left side, ferocity on the right and a sort of goodness in the middle. All round the room similar stories emerged – always the sadness on the left.

Jules explained a bit about the concept of right and left brain hemisphere functions. The right side of the brain which controls the left-hand side of the body seems to do with feelings, intuitions and a concept of 'the Whole', whereas the opposite combination controls action, critical analysis and understanding of 'the Particular'. Andrew commented that the chakra located on the brow is associated with laughter and fun! I didn't know any of this beforehand and felt it couldn't all be coincidence.

This brought us to a more general introduction to the chakra system.

The 'chakras' are bandied about these days as if everyone understood the term and as if they were as plain as the nose on your face. The concept is in fact borrowed from the ancient Tantric tradition of Hindu mysticism which began to gain favour among seekers of truth during the period of great interest in Eastern religions growing out of the hippy quest in the sixties, and which now is a feature of much modern mystical and holistic health thinking. It refers to a symbolic system of energy centres in the body ranged along the axis of the spine, corresponding roughly in our ordinary anatomical understanding to the location of the endocrine glands. Each one supposedly governs a different part of the body, different organs, glandular secretions, functions and emotions. If a blockage of energy flow occurs at any one of these junctions, disease, discomfort and malfunction are the result. Blockages are believed to be caused by negative thinking, unhealthy living, bad luck or bad 'karma'. (Karma is the celestial balance sheet of accrued credit and debit from previous incarnations. If you were wicked in a past life you may have to face the consequences in the present one. I still have a lot of trouble with the concept of reincarnation but I like the idea of being given the chance to make amends.)

The energy from the different chakras can be awakened and harmoniously balanced. The well-being of the physical body depends on this. They are charged by energy from the sun in the form of light which enters the chakras at different vibrationary rates causing each one to resonate to a different colour of the spectrum. All together they add up to the rainbow, the bridge between Man and God. I like that idea so much! A beautiful, simple symbol for harmony and change.

Chakra is the Sanskrit word for wheel. Skilled healers claim to be able to see great whirling catherine wheels of colour in these areas and can perceive if they are out of balance, deficient, or over-active. By visualizing therapeutic washes of the appropriate colour and focusing attention on the imbalances, the theory is that an ailing person can be brought back into harmony again – the energy balancing referred to in the description of this course.

Beginning at the base of the spine near the coccyx is the base or root chakra. It is the sexual and reproductive centre linked to the gonads and its colour is red.

At the junction with the pelvic bone is the abdominal or sacral chakra. It is linked to the adrenals, the active 'fight or flight' centre. It governs the kidneys and the digestive process and its colour is orange.

The solar plexus chakra is the yellow centre. It is linked to the rational intellectual left side of the brain. The pancreas is the gland in charge and it reflects disharmonies in the liver or spleen.

The heart chakra is our emotional centre. Green is its colour and it is in the area of the thymus. It reveals how we relate to people and how much 'heart' we put into things. Interestingly most people seem quite happy to accept this concept. The heart is well established in popular mythology as the place where we feel love or grief.

At the throat level is the blue centre. This takes care of communication, how we express ourselves and also the physical area of the neck and shoulders are vulnerable in this area. It is linked to the thyroid.

Violet is for the brow chakra, located in the region of the 'third eye', corresponding to the pituitary gland. This is the intuitive, non-verbal right side of the brain.

Finally right on the top of the head is the crown chakra, often depicted in Hindu or Buddhist painting as a thousand-petalled lotus flower. Linked to the pineal gland, this is our spiritual centre. From here we evolve our appreciation of art, religion and beauty, and connect with our concept of God. The colour is purple or white.

There are many smaller chakras all over the body but these main seven are the most important. It's a pretty abstract concept to try and get hold of, and easily falls into the trap of being taken too literally, but I thought it was a wonderful poetic and symbolic representation and a helpful aid to the visualization process.

Working in partners again we tried to explore and sense which areas radiated strongly and which seemed weak. At this stage I couldn't 'see' or sense any colours but I did actually feel a distinct coldness where her root chakra was supposed to be. When I looked up my notes later I realized that this is the area of sexuality and reproduction and Stella was indeed a rather dried-up middle-aged disappointed unmarried woman with a lot of regrets in her life. I tried to transmit healing in that spot. I was touched by a sweet desire on her part to give me something back in the way of affirmation. In that sense the healing is a very two-way process and this is where the self-healing comes in; the more you try to listen to others, the more you hear about yourself. The harder you look into the deep waters of another person's soul the more clearly you see your own reflection.

My dream that night was almost comical in its transparent symbolism. Andrew was the Wizard of Oz. He was actually called Oz and wore a cloak and a pointed hat with crescent moons and stars on it. Everyone was looking to him to be a magician so they could follow him and sit at his feet but he said he wasn't a proper magician at all. Just like in the film, when the travellers finally reached the Emerald City and there was no wizard. The lessons he had to teach were the things you learned on your journey to seek him.

'Seek and ye shall find,' said the wizard. 'Ask and it shall be given you. Knock and it shall be opened unto you.' And he gave me a gift of a lump of metal. I thought it was a worthless present and surreptitiously threw it away behind me but my son Tim was standing there and gave it back to me saying, 'Don't throw it away, it may be more valuable than you think.'

Jules pounced on this dream with glee, bringing up the legend of ancient alchemists turning base metal into gold, and how often in myths and fairy stories the homely old piece of junk turns out to be the real treasure (Aladdin's lamp, the cloak of invisibility, the magic carpet). It was interesting that I should receive this knowledge from the son I feel badly about not having been such a good mother to. I think my own areas of unease, remorse and shame are concerned with these guilty feelings about my failing Tim for a lot of his childhood. I've always admitted that and acknowledged it but rationalized it (he was a difficult baby, cried a lot, etc.). I think this time I've faced it honestly and have a genuine desire to make amends.

We did a long, guided meditation through a forest, meeting various symbolic objects along the way which, depending on how you pictured them, gave you some clues to the state of your masculine and feminine principles. This is basically derived from Jung's theory that we each have within us a set of traits and characteristics related to the opposite sex – our shadow aspects revealed in dream symbols that need to be recognized and integrated in order to attain the goals of maturity and harmonious balance. We didn't know this before we started though and were just to imagine ourselves in a forest. Mine was sunny and dappled, with giant redwood trees festooned with hanging moss like the rain forests of the north-west coast of America. I could see a lot of sparkling water in my mind's eye so when we were meant to come upon a lake, mine was there already. You find a chalice which you dip into the water and take on your way up a hill. Mine was a translucent pink onyx or alabaster goblet and the water I filled it with looked and tasted like mineral water, natural and effervescent. You come upon a sword. Mine seemed to be a heavy double-edged iron Crusader sword. King Richard the Lionheart was standing in the clearing and he handed it to me.

At the top of the hill you come to an altar and a priest is there (mine was a black monk) who won't tell you what to do but asks you to think what all these things mean to you. I wanted to drink the water and hang the sword on the wall. The altar seemed like my home and when we were meant to leave the forest and return, I felt I didn't need to travel anywhere.

The daydream seemed to be a cheerful image of wholeness and contentment, even bringing in Richard, my lionhearted husband, as the giver of my masculine principle. We had to share our experience in little groups and I was quite embarrassed to present my smug sunny fantasy when everyone else's in my group was so miserable. Poor Christopher had a bent, rusty sword and a cracked, leaky water pot – primitive, awkward, and too heavy to carry. The water all drained away and it was slimy and putrid anyway! One girl had a forest so dark and thick that she got totally lost. One had no water in the lake and a chalice that broke and crumbled when she tried to pick it up.

Finally, we discussed each other's symbols, attempting to cast some light on their significance and how a person might try to construct a model that they actually wanted to live up to, instead of hanging on to negative and self-destructive images. Then we divided into pairs and tried to give each other healing first from the masculine principle – holding the sword image in our minds; then from the feminine – holding the chalice image; and finally from a synthesis of both. Lynn and I sought each other out for this one, having not previously worked together before. She is a humorous, down-to-earth woman who also has a long-standing happy marriage and several kids. I wasn't terribly keen on the idea of a very unstable person messing around with my sexual balancing but once again intuition provided the right choice and we both enjoyed the experience. A few people got very upset and cried during this one. Poor Val, the young lesbian, went into terrible convulsions imagining a penis entering her. She was tenderly held by another woman until she fell asleep.

It was remarkable how people in the group had come to trust one another so fully that such hidden fears could be expressed in safety. There was so much love energy flowing – I had never felt it so strongly before anywhere. I began to believe that it really is a force that can move mountains.

At the end of the course we all felt immeasurably close to each other; forgiven and forgiving; understood and understanding. I felt both humbled and strengthened by what I learned. Maybe the most important lesson was that no one person had any more to give than anyone else. All had unique and very touching qualities. The need to give was more important and more healing than the need to receive. Receiving was far more difficult. The bonds between the group members became very strong, supportive and constructive. Very often those who felt they had been totally useless and inadequate at the healing exercises had testimonies to the contrary from their partners – they were giving a lot more than they knew.

The chakra areas really do seem to have some significance. Focusing healing energy on those specific points appears to bring dramatic results, and especially comfort, more quickly. I also learned that all healing is really self-healing – hence the name of this workshop – and that we each need to examine why we get ill, what we use illness for. What do the metaphors mean? Everyone was reluctant for the magic to end. We'd all brought wine and cheese and stayed on for a little celebration. Somebody played a concertina and somebody a country fiddle. Everyone danced and hugged, vowing to meet again come what may. It was hard to believe these powerful adventures had taken place over the course of only five days. 'Fear, not hate, is the opposite of love,' said Andrew.

I found to my amazement much later that images of stags, reindeer and other such creatures are very ancient symbols for regeneration and growth because of the way antlers are renewed. Antler symbolism goes back to Neolithic cave paintings and has been found in many parts of the world, often associated with the mysteries of death and rebirth.

Ever since I first embarked on this adventure, it became clear to me how treacherous are the quicksands that surround the subject of healing. There are so many rival factions. No one can agree on the interpretation of even the simplest word, and many potentially sympathetic listeners are easily antagonized or frightened off by bizarre claims and esoteric terminology. In a scientific age we are trying to deal with evidence that cannot be reconciled with science, with experiences that do not necessarily have rational explanations. Perhaps the biggest quagmire of all is the question of religious belief.

I have been a sort of open-minded agnostic all my life, delighted if something turns up, not too disappointed if it doesn't. As a child I was always conscious of a great deal of mystic activity and speculation going on in my mind but I didn't know how to describe it or define it and was reluctant to limit it by joining any one particular exclusive club which offered a package deal and claimed to have a monopoly on the truth. I was bewildered. All religions seemed to have something wonderful to offer; weren't they all pathways up the same mountain? Why did you have to choose? Supposing you made the wrong choice? Who were 'they' to claim to know they were right anyway and sit in judgement on the poor misguided fools who'd chosen wrongly? How dare they! No one can own God. I thought it then, and I still do.

For all this universal unconditional healing love energy to make any sense to me, I first had to be able to place it in an inter-denominational framework, so that when the word 'God' is used (and it's used a lot), it encompasses everybody's own personal interpretation.

> And almost everyone when age
> disease or sorrow strike him
> inclines to think there is a God
> or something very like him!

A living body is not a fixed thing but a flowing event, a flame, a whirlpool with no definite borders. The life force that animates us has to come from somewhere. To me the concept of God is simply the source of that energy: the infinite source of infinite power. Maybe it comes from within, maybe it comes from without, maybe the two are synonymous. With our brains' poor capacity to grasp the unimaginable, the infinite, the eternal, 'God' is just one of the many different poetic expressions we've invented in an attempt to capture the idea of the highest, the greatest, the ultimate. An attempt to find meaning and union with the world through full development of our specifically human capacities for love and reason.

Our great desire for certainty has led us to construct systems and dogmas around such fragments of knowledge and insight as we have perceived. What is common in the visions of different cultures has almost disappeared under the weight of misunder-standings between the various ideologies. And the bureaucrats, the rule-makers and the conformists that rise to the top in positions of power also have a vested interest in emphasizing the differences rather than that which is shared.

Words tend to add to the confusion. A concept can never adequately express the experience it refers to. It is, as the Zen Buddhists say, 'The finger that points to the moon.' It is not the moon.

There seems to be a lot of evidence that good health is involved with our spiritual natures and not solely a physical condition. I needed to explore this avenue more. The National Federation of Spiritual Healers is an old-established, well-respected organization so I went along to their 'Basic Healing Development Course' to see what I could learn. The Federation is founded on the premise that Man is a tri-unity of Body, Mind and Spirit, and that good health is a result of a harmonious balance between these three aspects.

In their definition, 'spiritual' doesn't have anything to do with spiritualism, which is the idea that departed spirits can communicate through a medium, but refers to the higher element and vibration in Man; the highest possible creative loving force. Through meditation, relaxation and concentration, a would-be healer tries to attune himself to these higher vibrations and make himself into a channel through which that force can travel. They don't claim to be discovering anything new, merely resurrecting something that has always been part of human experience – the tapping and using of a divine source of power, the power that is within us, in order to amplify the body's own healing gifts.

I realize that the desire to become good at something doesn't necessarily equate with ability. There are genius healers just as there are genius pianists and, although I may be able to meander through a Bach fugue after years of study, I will never be able to manage a Rachmaninov piano concerto or a Chopin scherzo – my hands aren't big enough and I don't have the dexterity. Just as I am not Ashkenazy I don't think I will ever be in the same league as those healers who have developed their psychic skills to the level of an art form. These people can apparently perceive in colour the magnetic energy fields that surround living bodies, they can influence the growth rate of seeds in a laboratory, they can leave their bodies and go astral travelling.

Most of us have lost this mental power, but luckily not entirely – it lies dormant and the object of the National Federation's courses and workshops is to teach the techniques that can help to develop and strengthen these extrasensory intuitive faculties into a set of tools we can use to keep our own bodies functioning well and to help us be jump leads for others.

There is just one more piano analogy before it gets tedious. Even if we don't possess a Steinway, we have no excuse for not keeping our humble instrument tuned. Impossible to play lovely music on a beat-up beer-stained honky-tonk, and you couldn't even play Chopsticks if the keys were missing and the strings broken. In the unlikely venue of an airport hotel conference room on the A4 near Heathrow, where the course was being held, we had lectures and discussions on ways to tune the instrument and opportunities to practise what we'd learned. One of the lecturers said, 'We are trying to link ourselves with the inexhaustible motive power that spins the universe.' Another interpreted it as 'God's healing power that flows through us'. I see it as trying to transcend the ego and leave behind the prison of one's selfishness and separateness.

Healers are dealing with a force which nobody really understands – a force that can disperse a growth, stimulate paralysed nerves, remove pain. As one spiritual healer said, 'No healer who has felt a misshapen spine straighten under his hand can doubt the power of this force. It is as potent as electricity and has to be used wisely.' 'Getting into the healing mode is an act of intention,' said another, reinforcing one of my first hunches. I must use my will to become receptive to the patient's needs and to become a conduit for energy. 'Alpha waves' is the name given to a particular pattern of brain waves which are produced when the state of being ready to heal is reached.

To try and achieve this state of stillness and calm we began with the simple act of breathing – something we all do approximately 23,000 times a day without giving it much thought. Being conscious of the breathing process and how to breathe correctly makes sense to me and I like the poetic and mystical concept of breath as the vitality of the universe. More than the mere inhalation of chemicals, prana, the Sanskrit word for breath, also means 'soul'. It is an airborne magic, the essence that affects consciousness. Control of the breath, directing its beneficial properties to parts of the body, slowing it down to deep gentle rhythm, precedes relaxation and opens the way for dynamic changes to take place.

A healer is useless to anyone else until he has made a start at putting his own house in order, and with that first commitment of learning to use the power of the mind creatively in order to bring about changes I felt I was consciously taking responsibility for my own physical and mental well-being. I am neither omnipotent nor helpless. I can walk in step with myself, with others and with the universe. It was an affirmation of my power and an awakening of it.

I am acutely aware that, as a would-be healer, I must be wary of the traps lying in wait. Ego trips? Saviour complex? Rescue fantasies? Who do I think I am, wanting to be a healer? Do I have ulterior motives of my own? Unmet needs? What business is it of mine to want to intervene? So saying, and whilst recognizing the ever-present dangers and inherent pitfalls, I feel that false modesty would also be inappropriate. I know I have skills with energy. I can raise it and cause it to flow. What I want to learn is how to apply and direct it. This is where visualization comes in again. Just visualizing the process of the diaphragm muscle contracting and expanding, causing the lungs to fill with air then forcing them to expel it, seems to focus the attention on what's happening. I pictured the air whooshing through my limbs as though they were hollow macaroni, as though I were inhaling and exhaling through my fingers and toes, through all the orifices of my body. Deep, even, life-giving breaths, calming my mind, slowing my metabolic rate, refreshing my body, leading me into a state of relaxation – the Alpha state. This is a very receptive condition where you are fully conscious but have opened a channel to the intuitive creative part of your mind. From this point it's often quite tempting to go to sleep.

If that is what you need, go ahead and do it, advised the course leader; otherwise you can move into the state of meditation where you attempt to clear your mind of all distracting thoughts. I'm not very good at this and most people I've talked to seem to find it difficult to begin with. As soon as I try to think of nothing, every trivial detail of the day's events springs instantly to mind and washes about like sewage in the forefront of my brain. Boring pieces of information for which I now have total recall buzz drearily round and round like fat bluebottles on a summer afternoon.

Repeating a mantra as an aid to concentration, counting my breaths, or imagining nothing but a bright yellow sun filling my mind, helped me to push other thoughts away. I persevered and managed to get a bit better at it, markedly so when in the company of a group of others striving for the same goal. The combined efforts of several willing souls always seem greater than the sum of their parts – rather like singing in a choir. You get a tremendous lift-off and feel as if you are soaring on eagle's wings.

I first got interested in this type of meditation about ten years ago. I was impressed by my friend Kay's remarkable serenity and good humour despite the fact that she had four children, was studying for a degree in education and was married to a boorish man who used to hit her, hide the car keys and tear up her essays during his pathetic jealous tantrums. Quite simply, meditation gave her the strength and conviction to carry on. I admired her so much and persuaded her to take me along to the Study Society where she had learned the technique.

A very generous and altruistic spirit prevailed there. I was assigned to someone who would monitor my progress and whom I could contact if I had any problems. Everything was done out of kindness and love and no money was asked for. After a couple of months I participated in a simple ritual ceremony with candles and flowers and my mantra was given to me.

I'm sorry to say I lapsed shamefully, after an initial burst of enthusiasm, although I really got a lot out of it. I don't know why I didn't keep it up. Perhaps because trying to find any peace and quiet in a houseful of noisy children made me more tense and frustrated than if I hadn't bothered, and partly because I wasn't quite ready for the introspection. Looking back I can see that it was a significant step for me because it marked the first time I'd seriously considered marshalling my internal forces in order to become less of a victim to chance and circumstance. The first time I'd tried to bring the vehicle into contact with the driver.

This time with my children grown up and more time to think, I was ready for it and found the lessons of those early days very useful. This type of meditation is a great solvent of stress and gives the body's self-healing mechanism an opportunity to recover its authority. I always feel better when I make time to do it; intellectual and spiritual changes seem to take place enabling me to see things and problems in a new light, with a new awareness. The unveiling is more likely to happen when the quiet side of the mind is given a chance. As one of the lecturers said, 'A brick would not be noticed thrown on to a turbulent sea but a pebble will be noticed on a quiet pond.'

The other type of meditation is really a sort of guided day-dreaming such as I learned with Andrew Watson – I suspect it's what imaginative kids do all the time until they're bullied out of it by adults telling them to stop wasting time. They are exercising the mind's marvellous image-making capacity and projecting themselves into places and situations where they'd rather be. 'Miles away,' we say. 'Off in a world of his own.'

One of the greatest and most astonishing feats of the human

mind is the ability to visualize, to evoke images seemingly from nowhere. As a simple example, while pondering on the daunting nature of my self-appointed mission to try and pick a plain woman's path through this complex maze, my mind suddenly conjured up a picture of myself standing alone on the edge of the Arctic Ocean. In front of me were thousands of ice floes stretching into infinity. They were easy stepping stones but I had no way of telling which ones would bear my weight or which ones would flip over leaving me floundering in the icy water, or sweep me off my course and disintegrate out of sight of land while I sank without trace! Of course we make metaphors in dreams all the time, as if the subconscious mind is a library of cross-references and just in case you haven't got the point, it will think up another image to clarify it. It's as if you knew it all along and the revelation is merely uncovering what is within, connecting with the source of wisdom. 'I see!' we cry; 'I get the message'; 'I understand'. You suddenly know something. Where does that knowledge come from? God? The higher self? The 'universal unconscious'? I am content that it is there and that I occasionally make contact with it.

I want to tell the story of one of those rare moments where the truth seemed just within reach. Most of us get these illuminations from time to time. 'Ah hah!' I said to myself at the time. I also know that, as when someone tries to describe a powerful experience under the influence of mind-expanding drugs, it does sound a bit mad to anyone who hasn't shared the sensations. Here goes anyway.

I was staying in Devon with old friends, Adam and Jo. We'd all been struggling a bit in the recent past with various personal dilemmas and were grateful for the friendship as a balm and mutual support system. We climbed one day to the top of Brentor in the middle of Dartmoor. A thirteenth-century church stands on this ancient site. It is a landmark visible for miles around, rugged and steadfast with an enchanted atmosphere. It was February and a fierce wind blew, snow swirled around us as we opened the gates of the church at the top and went in. The little church is peaceful, and cherished; still in use, with fresh flowers and stained-glass windows transforming the thin winter light to a warm glow. But I felt strangely that the forces of power were actually not inside the building and experienced a strong desire to go back outside where the wind was howling and the hail and snow driving across the moor in gusty sweeping gales, knocking me off my feet and buffeting me furiously. I made my way around the outside of the church, hanging on for dear life to the guard rail to prevent myself being blown off the mountain until I reached the side that was sheltered from the wind and magically still in the midst of the turbulent weather raging round about.

There is a little seat facing out across the rolling moors and I sat down. Adam and Jo came out and found me and we sat together. Suddenly right in front of us the sun appeared strong and bright and warm on our faces sending down slanting rays like those pictures in a child's illustrated Bible: 'Where two or three are gathered together in my name, I will be among you.' When there is a desire and longing for the light of truth, then the combined power of two or three minds genuinely and humbly seeking enlightenment will be blessed by the grace of 'God', which I saw then as a glinting crystal with many facets shining in the sunlight before us.

I mentioned what I was thinking to the others and Adam looked quite shaken. Just before I'd spoken, he said, he'd clearly seen standing before us the white-robed figure of Christ who said 'My blessings are with you' and faded. I thought it was so interesting that we both had had an experience of equal intensity and of identical content – only the mind pictures had been different, conditioned by our personal beliefs. We stayed a while then descended the hillside quite certain that our friendship – that coincidental yet somehow inevitable link with one another – was a way forward through our current crises to a higher plane of understanding, purpose and resolution.

I learned on this National Federation course that 'Christ consciousness' is quite a common vision through meditation, a projection of a higher manifestation from the mind's attempt to give birth to something beautiful. It might be an explanation of the intense visions of the saints described in Christian folklore.

How marvellous that, as fellow humans, we can be united in a common goal — believers and non-believers alike — for which actions, not concepts, give us clues about each other, about the human reality behind the thought.

Visualization is one of the healer's most powerful tools, so learning to develop and use it is of primary importance. There's nothing mystical about this. When I plant bulbs in my garden in the autumn, I visualize the carpet of crocuses in spring. It's merely a projection onto your mental cinema screen of what you want to see. We did exercises with all the senses, using our imaginations to conjure up in detail a flower so clearly that the petals could be counted, the feel of tree bark, the texture of velvet, the smell of jasmine, the taste of lemon, the sound of an oboe.

You begin to enter into an altered state where the distinctions between the physical and the imaginary become less clearly defined. If your teeth can be set on edge by the thought of a fingernail scraped on a blackboard, if your mouth can water at the thought of a Marmite sandwich, if you can become sexually aroused by erotic fantasies, that mental power can be harnessed. And if you can accept, as I do, that the mind plays a very creative part in the formation of disease, so it follows that the mind can play an equally creative part in its eradication — lowering blood pressure, relieving pain, relaxing tensions. I feel even more certain that good health is not solely a question of physical condition.

After these preliminary warm-up exercises we practised a simple visualization. First of all the deep breathing, the state of relaxation, the preparation for meditation, then one of the lecturers set the scene: you are standing in a narrow country lane heavy with the scents of summer hedgerows and the sounds of birdsong. Warm breezes ruffle your hair and the sun feels delicious on your skin. You climb over a stile and walk across the meadows and cornfields full of poppies. You chew on a straw, you lie by a pond, you dangle your fingers in the water . . .

It is a wonderful way to develop your concentration and imagination and to cultivate the habit of travelling beneath the surface. Instead of worrying like demented sheep pursued by stray dogs, we can learn the art of sustained reflection. Concentration focuses the enormous power of the mind like a magnifying glass. For me, this is certainly a very fruitful area for self-improvement. I am learning not to be governed by hasty, superficial and misleading appearances. Most of us are so busy with what goes on on the outside that we are unaware of the miraculous imaginative complexity going on inside.

'Don't let's dull this vital force,' says John Dreghorn, one of the lecturers. 'It is the very thing that brings about the state of attunement where the mind can become the willing servant of the higher self.' Healing is a natural, law-abiding process. 'Wounds will close, blood will clot, toxic substances will be expelled all by themselves under normal circumstances.' All a healer does is to present himself, a willing channel for the divine spark, so to speak, to the patient's higher self. Then what the patient does with it is up to him; if the disease has fulfilled its purpose it will go away.

Sometimes getting better is not the outcome. Healing is not synonymous with cure but can also be seen as the process of letting go. Death is not necessarily a failure. Healers should be careful not to impose their need to see results or ever try to cultivate dependence. We are just a support system, a set of jump leads. The only person who can heal a patient is, ultimately, himself.

We did a little practical work on each other just to get our hands in, as it were. Using the palms of the hands, beginning at the head and working slightly away from the body you scan the chakras for any sensation of imbalance. Then, by whichever visualization you feel comfortable with, you focus your beam of energy on the needy area. That's it, in a nutshell. The Federation is keen to dispel the broomstick image of healing and warn against the dangers of healers seeing themselves as an elite. They disapprove of tricksy mannerisms, funny voices, props and accoutrements. Why go into a trance and hand over responsibility to another authority? Their objective is to transcend the intermediary 'spirit guides' who communicate through mediums, and reach the higher self, confident in its own inner knowledge.

That is our birthright, our natural unifying force as human beings – inter-denominational and undogmatic.

I thought they were sane, normal people doing a damn good job and I have joined the Federation as a probationary member. They have a sensible code of ethics emphasizing the importance of working alongside the medical profession, never attempting to diagnose nor to dissuade patients from taking their prescribed medication. We are extremely fortunate in Great Britain that the law allows practitioners of alternative medicine considerable freedom and we must be careful never to give anyone cause to regret it. John Dreghorn told the story of a healer who claimed that the 'Force' didn't travel through nylon and would the young lady please remove her blouse! There will probably always be weirdos and perverts trying to cash in on a situation ripe for exploitation. The Federation is trying to work out an effective monitoring system that doesn't cramp the individual's healing style and yet offers the consumer some reassurance of competence.

2

The Imprisoned Splendour

I had never heard of the work of Elisabeth Kübler-Ross until I saw a BBC television interview with her about a year ago and was enormously moved by her humanity and wisdom. Here was a woman with a lot to say about healing. She is a medical doctor and a psychiatrist, who for many years has pledged her skills to working with terminally ill patients – helping them and their relatives to come to terms with death.

The greatest barrier, as she sees it, to a peaceful acceptance of death – or life, come to that – is the weighty crushing burden of unfinished business we all carry around with us. We are still tormented by fears when there is no reason to be afraid. We fuel old resentments and drown in the unshed tears of buried grief. In the words of Piero Ferrucci, 'We hang on to the ticket long after we have left the bus.'

This kind of negativity is exhausting and destructive but when the patterns that force us to such useless expenditures of energy are confronted they lose their potency, and when they are shared in the safety of a caring group they are exposed for what they are – repressed or misdirected natural emotions which have gone sour, causing us to become a bundle of anxieties, phobias and doubts, ruining our potential for growth and happiness, making us afraid of life and afraid of death.

To this end Dr Ross began her Life, Death and Transition workshops. She wanted to create a safe environment of mutual support where dying patients could deal with their unfinished business, come to terms with their anguish, terror and bewilderment and try to make some sense of it.

She found that many of these patients expressed the thought that we are all in the same boat really, with 'x' days to live, only they have been given an additional poignant gift – the opportunity to cherish their remaining days and use them well. The finite nature of life is actually a blessing in disguise, for it isn't the quantity of life that counts but the quality. The proximity of death reminds us to make the most of life, to live each day as if it is the last one we have.

Clearly, these lessons can be learned at any stage of life's journey and the dying patients proved to be the best teachers of all, so now the workshops are extended to include almost anyone who wants to participate. They are held all over the world in the name of Elisabeth Kübler-Ross's foundation, Shanti Nilaya, and consist of about one-third health care professionals – doctors, nurses, healers, counsellors – one-third dying patients and one-third bereaved relatives – parents of children who have committed suicide, parents of murdered children, people consumed by agony and pain. They come together to learn, to share, to let go and to grow in an atmosphere of unconditional love and unqualified acceptance: true healing indeed.

I knew I would learn a lot from participating in one of these five-day workshops so I wrote requesting a place on the next one, to be held fortuitously in England.

I had a dream once, of mercury. A broken thermometer scattered myriad silver pearls everywhere. Like the Milky Way, a thousand droplets – all perfect spheres in their own right – raced across the galaxy, winking and tumbling in the moonlight – but they fused seamlessly when pushed together to form one shining flawless fluid globe.

It seemed deeply symbolic of an intrinsic desire common to all organic life to belong to a larger whole – a beautifully graphic representation of our collective unconscious. A longing for oneness which is by no means an obliteration of individual uniqueness or a negation of personal responsibility, but merely the opposite of an icy void, the antithesis of isolation.

The week started with a room full of separate little silver balls.

A random rush-hour tube train full of odds and ends of human beings, each with their prejudices, bravados and fears – making small talk on the outside and instant judgement on the inside. What coincidence or divine manipulation had brought us together to a quiet retreat in the Kent countryside? What common destiny found us here with this extraordinary little woman?

Elisabeth, as she likes to be called, is a small grey sparrow with specs too big for her face – a sublime face she has earned by the life that she lives, warm and kind and etched with laughter. A beatific face of compassion and wisdom. She sits on a chair with her shoes off and her knees drawn up under her chin, her head cocked to one side and her body leaning forward in an attitude of intense concentration, alertness and responsiveness. She speaks in a quiet voice as if to conserve her strength. She does not waste words but has that great ability of gifted teachers to illuminate in anecdotes and stories, with humour and pathos, a seam of purest gold that shines with the simplicity of truth. You know you are in the presence of someone who has made a leap of understanding and perceived the interconnectedness of all things. She is refreshingly unmeek, a practical Swiss with a strong character, a mischievous sense of humour and a healthy instinct to protect her own needs from the voraciousness of others.

Because she is doing what she loves and her motivation is of the highest calibre, she appears to draw on a superhuman energy. She cheerfully acknowledges that divine helpers, guardian angels, or 'spooks' as she calls them come to her rescue when she has exhausted her own resources. She simply accepts and is grateful for the little miracles that come her way and the spiritual intuitions and revelations that allow her transcendental glimpses of the other side. That energy is the very source of her conviction and strength and enables her to work eighteen hours a day, seven days a week, with dying children, with AIDS sufferers, with a couple who lost all their children from cancer within six months, with a mother whose little girl was eaten by sharks, and still retain her hope and optimism.

Her faith is clearly the framework of her existence but she is careful never to label it nor to preach, avoiding the divisiveness of conflicting ideological dogma. She sees the differences in beliefs and mythologies as merely interesting cultural variations since the essential truth is common to all religions and accessible to everyone by whichever pathway. Differences are to be respected, not eradicated.

In the meantime she spends her life not with esoteric theories about higher cosmic consciousness but with healing human beings very much here on the ground. When caring for dying patients she stresses that it is absolutely imperative to attend to their physical needs above all else, as you would a child in the first year of life. They must be pain-free and conscious and in a loving environment, preferably at home with children around them and music and maybe a favourite animal. Only then can you help them take care of their emotional needs, their unfinished business.

The healing itself is very simple and anyone can do it; the only requirement is fully to appreciate what you have and get rid of the negativity that blocks you from becoming whole. Healing in our time is to do with openness. When you have the humility to open yourself you can reach this inner knowledge and allow your intuition and understanding to speak.

'You cannot heal anyone else without healing yourself,' says Elisabeth. 'You cannot heal the world without healing the child inside of you.'

This is the diary I kept during that extraordinary week. A week which turned out to be largely about 'owning' your feelings, gaining access, taking possession and acknowledging responsibility. Once you fully own something you can choose whether you want to keep it or throw it away. You can't help what has been done to you but you can choose whether or not you want to be a victim forever.

It seemed suddenly clear to me that what Jesus meant by 'turning the other cheek' was not passive complicity and resignation but active choice – the choice not to be a victim but to exercise forgiveness and responsibility. Even *in extremis* this symbolic gesture would rob another human being from ever having ultimate power over you. It would even rob death of its victory, for you become indestructible. Death is not the enemy but the final stage of growth.

Monday 10 September

As I write this I have such a thudding pounding headache I can hardly think straight. For two or three days before coming on this workshop I have been brewing up some dreadful tension which I can't interpret. I hope it will become clear over the course of the next few days. Elisabeth, when I asked her, said that when I've released whatever it is that's bothering me the headache will go. I didn't come here thinking I had very much work to do on myself. I arrogantly feel pretty well adjusted without too much unfinished business of my own to attend to. Maybe I have some surprises in store.

We assembled in the conference hall and arranged ourselves in a big circle, some of us on chairs, some sitting about on mattresses on the floor. One of Elisabeth's assistants has a little guitar – and we begin the proceedings with a couple of songs. My heart sinks. I am quite resistant to this as I don't like jolly singalongs much and I hate songs like 'This little light of mine', although strangely enough the one they chose to start with, 'You are my sunshine', does have heart-tugging childhood significance for me – I used to be made to sing it in my piping three-year-old's voice to cheer people up in the air-raid shelters during the Blitz. And I have to acknowledge the fact that singing does create a feeling of mutual endeavour and raises a high level of natural energy. The choice of songs will never please everybody so I force myself to join in the spirit of the thing.

Then everyone in the group one by one stands and introduces themselves. A few words about why you are here and what you think is your greatest strength and your greatest weakness. This is a very clever starting manœuvre as everyone is forced immediately to own up to something they don't like about themselves and credit themselves with something positive. I say that I am here because I feel I am on a journey of discovery, that my greatest

43

weakness is impatience and my greatest strength a capacity for happiness.

We are a large group – about seventy people – so this takes a long time. I am surprised that Elisabeth likes to work with such large numbers. At the moment it seems unwieldy but the little brief introductions are very interesting – some very moving in their stark simplicity. Already the instant judgements are beginning to seem uncharitably rash and shamingly inaccurate. There are several cancer patients, nurses, doctors, social workers, counsellors, and many people suffering recent bereavements – a mother whose son committed suicide, a husband whose young wife was killed by medical negligence, a girl who lost both her parents in a car crash. People appear to be honestly trying to find their reasons for being here but perhaps, like me, many don't really know.

Next we all repair to the dining-room and are given a quick fifteen minutes to do a drawing of anything that comes to mind using a variety of coloured crayons. Elisabeth believes that a great deal of useful diagnostic and preventive work can be done from the interpretation of drawings as they spring like dreams from what she calls the intuitive spiritual quadrant of the mind, bypassing the intellect and revealing areas that need attention. Even if you try, it's very difficult to fool yourself. The choice of each colour has significance, although we didn't know that until afterwards: red for anger, pain, fear and hurt; orange for change; yellow for energy; black for grief; brown for health and harmony; green for photosynthesis and growth; blue for healing, balance and wholeness; white means desperately trying to hide something – a reluctance to reveal your true self.

Significance can also be read in the choice of the symbols themselves, the brightness or faintness of the colours, the variety and number of objects, and positioning of the layout. The lower left-hand quarter of the picture is to do with the past, the lower right-hand quarter to do with the immediate future, the upper left-hand quarter is the far future and the upper right-hand quarter the present. So much can be read into it if you know what to look for but, as with any tool of course, enthusiastic misuse by amateurs can do more harm than good. We are warned of the dangers. My picture was an enormous blue bird flying through orange rain towards a bright red-orange sun in the upper left-hand corner (future). There was a deep-rooted brown tree in the lower left-hand corner (past), a black tulip in the immediate future and bright flowers in groups of three springing out of green hills in the foreground.

Everyone's was amazingly different, of course: a black house with tiny windows high up where no one could see in; a house with a pathway leading up but not to the front door; a tree with no roots only half on the page; a pair of huge eyes staring; a volcano erupting with red lava; one that just said 'NO WAY' in heavy black letters.

We spent the rest of the evening analysing a number of them. Very intriguing how the archetypal symbols keep on cropping up – being good or terrible at drawing didn't make any difference. Anyone who didn't get theirs read could ask for an interpretation later. I still don't quite understand how you can tell the difference between what is really a hot-line to the truth and what is an anxious projection of fear, or tell when people are merely latching on to what's expected of them. Maybe it doesn't matter – it's all part of you just the same. All the while my headache becomes more excruciating and I have resorted to painkillers, but it still won't go away.

Tomorrow we get down to business. Some people here are old campaigners who have been on a lot of courses – EST, Esalen, Findhorn, etc, searching for a way to deal with the repressed feelings they carry around inside. Elisabeth, after many years of experience and experiment, believes that only in these very large groups is it possible to cover ground so quickly. With thirty people it would take five weeks, she says. Because of the range of emotions brought to the group by such large numbers, if somebody starts to have an abreactive experience it will trigger responses all around the room. 'More people to push your buttons,' as she puts it.

I went for a long jog/walk out across the golden late summer fields at 7 am this morning before breakfast. Sitting cramped in the conference room all day may be good for the soul but it is not good for the body: I was dying for some exercise. The countryside looked lovely – benign and mellow. I devoured the fresh air greedily and ate some hedgerow blackberries.

We began today's workshop, after the sing-song, with a discussion about the five natural emotions and how they become twisted into their unnatural perverted forms. These are the enemy within that we are out to defuse so it is important to recognize them that they may be unmasked and disarmed.

Anger is a natural emotion. Its purpose is change and in its normal state it shouldn't last more than about 15 seconds. If it is repressed it turns into rage, revenge, self-destructiveness, hate and depression. Public enemy number one.

Fear – of only two things – loud noises and falling – is a natural emotion. Its purpose is survival. In its unnatural form it becomes anxiety, phobia, panic.

Grief serves the vital purpose of resolving losses. When denied a healthy outlet it turns into self-pity, depression, shame and guilt.

Jealousy triggers emulation and therefore evolution. When it gets out of proportion it becomes envy, greed, competitiveness, manipulation and hypocrisy.

Love, that makes the world go round and bonds us together, can turn to prostitution, possessiveness, a pathetic need for approval and a lack of confidence.

The patterns of these mangled emotions go back to childhood every time, of course, when we were told 'Big boys don't cry'; 'Don't be a sissy'; 'I'll love you if you behave yourself/get good marks/do as you're told'; 'Buck up, you're a soldier's daughter'; 'Shut up crying or I'll give you something to cry about.'

All this talk created a climate where bottled-up feelings began to well up and people started to come forward spontaneously one at a time to share their troubles. There is a mattress at the front covered by a fitted sheet and on it are a stack of old phone books and a length of rubber hose. This is for beating out your suppressed anger, rage and disappointment. Elisabeth, by careful listening and an unerring knack of picking up the relevant thread, gently gets the person to follow it up and to project the objects of hate or fury on to the telephone books, howl out the pent-up misery in a torrent of verbal abuse and beat the hell out of them with the rubber hose. Old grief dissolves in a deluge of tears and there is a pillow for hugging and talking to. Guilt and remorse relinquish their grip by confession and self-forgiveness. Screaming gets your initial fears up from the depths of your bowels and helps you recognize them for what they are.

It's very distressing and humbling to listen to all these chronicles of pain. A mother whose teenage son died from a drug overdose. A young man whose beautiful mother left him as a baby when she had a schizophrenic breakdown and was put in a mental institution and given shock treatment. She came home all changed, irrational and unpredictable. Then she died when he was fifteen and he's never resolved his grief and loss and sense of betrayal. There was a woman who wanted to, and nearly did, poison her unfaithful husband; the poor man whose wife died as a result of a mistake by a nurse after a simple routine operation – he shook and shook as he relived it and strangled the hosepipe to death with his bare hands. A vicar's son, a respectable middle-aged accountant, rushed up to the front and wrote 'FUCK The God People' on the board and beat up his parents and boarding-school teachers and raged against them all for telling him that God was Love while he saw the hypocrisy and suffered the sadism of their miserable dishonest lives. 'Thank you,' he said quietly to all of us when he'd finally spent himself. 'I've wanted to do that all my life but never dared.'

Elisabeth has explained that at this stage it is not helpful to try and comfort anyone. There will be time enough for that later. Right now it is important for the catharsis to take place uninterrupted. It is also important to notice in yourself which stories really upset you because that is often the key to your own unfinished business.

The size of this huge group seems to have more significance now. It's small enough (just) for you to be surrounded by people you know are here for the same purpose, yet large enough for your 'confession' to seem public in a meaningful way. You've revealed deeply hidden things in front of strangers and you don't feel ashamed or foolish because no one is judging you. The audience are all compassionate and you are accepted by them for what you really are. You are also accepted by that which is greater than you – call it what you will – it is not dependent on religious belief. Acceptance is the beginning of growth.

All the while Elisabeth listens and follows and waits, never losing the scent of the trail. 'Tell your mother what it felt like when she left you.' 'Tell your father what terror you went through when he came home drunk and violent.' 'Project yourself on to the phone books, tell yourself what you don't like about you.'

If someone in the listening circle becomes distraught and starts to react very strongly to something being enacted while the mattress is already occupied, or if it seems as if a person will blossom better in private, they go off to a side room with one of the assistants.

Elisabeth tells her own stories too, her old unfinished business now laid to rest. How as an obedient Swiss child she was made to take her silky black pet bunny rabbit, her love object, to the butchers and bring back the still-warm package of meat for the Sunday roast; the misery of being an identical triplet whom not even her parents could tell apart from her sisters.

I sit and listen. To be honest, I am alternately deeply touched and somewhat fidgety. A few people's sagas seem a little shopworn, if that's not too cruel; they tend to cry a lot and hog the floor – you get the feeling that workshops have become a way of life. They follow them round the world like a little herd of grazing herbivores looking for green pastures.

Nothing, so far, has made me want to share a thing. I honestly feel my own happy childhood that gave me the ability to form loving relationships has me on a pretty stable footing. Perhaps I do have a Hitler to face somewhere but I'm not sure this is my way. I don't sense any skeletons in my cupboards. The only time

I had a slight welling up of emotion was thinking about my father's pain in his life – the tragedy of the decimation of his family and the weight of Jewish grief he carried around until he died. It probably even contributed to his fatal cancer. Maybe I'd like to shed some tears for him.

We had breaks for meals but went on till way after midnight. It's hot and cramped and uncomfortable in the hall and I still feel something needs to happen to pull this thing properly together, to avoid the danger of loosing all these fireworks, lighting all these touchpapers without the time or the individual care to complete the unfinished business.

Wednesday 12 September

It really is extraordinary how people will suddenly feel moved to shed their burdens. One after another the most unlikely people come forward prepared to tell their stories in front of the group. I was particularly touched by Annie from New Zealand: a neat, efficient, brisk, perfectionist nurse who works as a bereavement counsellor. She followed swiftly after a woman who'd wept and raged about her husband's infidelity but decided to stick with him anyway. Annie suddenly blew up about bloody, fucking, cowardly women who can't be anything without a bloody man and out poured the story of her own mother – simpering, pretty and helpless. Abandoned by her first husband, she had married again and left for England, taking the children without telling them they were going for good. Altogether Annie had had four 'fathers' in her life but none of them stayed. Men had always let her down except the one she was now married to and she was afraid she would drive him away if she didn't learn to love him and trust him in time. Last night she had dreamed about him in a garden of roses. 'It's the first time I've ever had the right man in the right place at the right time,' she said. 'I want to get rid of my old conditioning and love him the way he deserves.'

A brassy blonde grandmother from South Africa was next. Rather gushy and a bit irritating – her story nevertheless really taught me a lot. She was the tenth of eleven children raised on a farm and never remembered sitting on her mother's lap. Every morning after her dad got up she used to try and get into bed with her mum but one of the others always beat her to it. Her mum never moved over to make room for her and she was forever falling off the edge. She cried and cried about her desolate loneliness and longing for physical affection. Her voice was that of a three-year-old. When she'd finished, Elisabeth cleared the mattress of all the torn-up phone books and said, 'Now you're going to have that whole bed.' The woman lay down and everyone in the group linked arms to make a living cradle and rocked her like a little child, singing 'Swing Low, Sweet Chariot'. There were lots of tears and lots of hugging suddenly. Many gulfs were bridged and hands reached out to touch other hands. A perfect example of unconditional love. You could feel the thrum of healing energy binding everyone together. The will of the group had brought that power into the room and it was all focused on this little, middle-aged woman that normally you'd probably avoid at the office party but that suddenly you could see completely non-judgementally and with total compassion.

It made me very tearful – I don't know if it touched something specific in me, but I felt very much in awe of the power I could feel, also tremendously conscious of the responsibility of handling these confessions if you're in Elisabeth's shoes. When do you suggest working it out in private? When do you encourage more screaming and banging? When do you know a person has finished for the time being and when to probe for more? When does their body language or tone of voice tell you something?

Elisabeth says she enters a state of intense concentration where she becomes very tuned into the person and their needs. 'Then if you can stop thinking for a change,' she says, 'allow your intuition to speak and do what comes to you without judging and criticizing, you have a chance to heal him.'

One woman with cancer who had lost her brother and sister from the same disease talked about her terror of dying. Elisabeth immediately suggested she did a series of drawings visualizing her cancer, the alternative therapies that could be tried and also her image of 'wholeness'. She believes a patient invariably knows at a subconscious level more about their illness and the type of treatment it will best respond to than is generally recognized.

The challenge of this workshop is to be able to face the future with confidence and self-determination no matter what has gone before or no matter how short a time you have left.

My big shock came when I finally got Elisabeth to read my drawing during the lunch break. I had felt rather smugly that it was pretty healthy – bright sun, big bird, tree with roots. But . . . she took one look at it and said, 'Why is your bird flying backwards?' Apparently my choice of faded baby-blue indicates very faint confidence.

I am trying to nest my huge unconfident bird in the little brown tree of my childhood. The tree itself, though strongly rooted with much growth, has very disconnected branches and no leaves. My tulip, although it has a green fertile stem, also has a big black flower of grief. My sun is a burning red holocaust of pain and anger overlaid and intermingled with a lot of orange, signifying change. The bird is flying through nineteen huge orange rain drops (could be tears) and numbers always mean something (the age I was when my first child was born and my own childhood ended?).

The whole thing has made me feel a bit flaky, as the Americans would say. I can't really understand either the anger or the grief to be anything I need to get in touch with – although the headache I have had all week still persists – they are both areas I think I have faced and worked well on: the roller coaster of a long-standing, impassioned and creative marriage with its hot-blooded issues of give and take, jealousies and compromises – I really think I have expressed all those emotions in a safe framework. The anger but also the progress and the healing are there.

I also feel I grieved properly when my mum died recently. I was honest about the anger and sorrow I felt by what I perceived as her wilful self-destruction and yet again proud and touched by her enormous capacity to love and her courage to do things her way.

I do feel shaken though – maybe it's just being in the presence of so much raw emotion.

After lunch, about the second person to come forward was a

German woman. She had a whole bunch of stuff to do with her father – anger and rejection – that she was trying to work out, but the English language wasn't giving her the words she needed to tap the source.

Elisabeth, who of course speaks German, said, 'Speak to him in your own language.' So she started beating the phone books and screaming in German – a rising crescendo of rabid fury – and suddenly, without any warning, up from the bottom of my well came a surging force like vomit. My heart broke into a gallop, the blood pounded in my head, my breathing quickened and my whole body started to tremble.

Just as soon as Helga had exhausted herself I was on that mattress before I knew what had happened. The terrible sound of all that beating and German shouting had detonated my unexploded bomb of ancient grief about my gentle daddy and his aching sorrow over the loss of his family, his language, his people.

All the pain of his pain, I had never allowed myself to endure when I was a child because I couldn't bear to see my mother's distress when she tried to tell me about it. She wanted me to understand why he sometimes wept and had nightmares. She tried to tell me the Germans had killed little children and thrown live babies into ovens and beaten old people to death. Tears welled in her eyes as she spoke and her voice would catch in her throat. I used to stick my fingers in my ears and refuse to listen; I'd run out of the room and scream 'Don't tell me!'

When I got older and reached my teens I knew that I would have to try and face it of my own accord sooner or later so I read *The Diary of Anne Frank* and a couple of harrowing accounts of what went on in the concentration camps, but I could never ask my father to tell me about it because I didn't know how to deal with the enormity of adult grief.

Once I learned some Yiddish folk songs to sing him because I thought it would make him happy but he sobbed and sobbed like a baby and I was powerless to comfort him.

Now all I wanted to do was to tell him I knew and I understood and I loved him. That he didn't need to feel guilty for having survived when they died because his life had been worth living. The suffering had not been in vain and the love that he gave transcended all the evil; it was a beacon that still shines on his children and his children's children.

So I picked up the pillow and held him in my arms and said it all and cried those tears I'd held in for so long. I hardly knew where I was or what I was doing. I was oblivious to the seventy people in the room where my black tulip had bloomed and as I gradually stopped rocking and swaying and tenderly laid the pillow down I heard Elisabeth's voice say, 'Thank you, you've pushed a lot of people's buttons.'

Half the people around me were crying and a whole new phase of reactions was sparked off. At last I understand how the chemistry works.

The next person to come forward was another German woman. (What kind of coincidence is it that brought the three of us here to this English group?) She picked up the truncheon and bashed and bashed screaming, 'It wasn't my fault, it wasn't my fault – I was only a baby.' Then she spoke like a zombie in a small dead voice saying that she was ashamed and frightened to tell the group the worst thing about her. Elisabeth waited, we all waited, until she blurted out that she was a Nazi officer's daughter. He'd been a good father and she'd loved him. Now ten years after his death she was trying to disentangle the feelings she had for a loving father from her abhorrence of his wartime role.

There was also the confusion of her own anti-Semitic childhood indoctrination – still a legacy of conditioned reflexes after all these years.

We looked into each other's eyes in bewilderment and pain. A horrible tangle of barbed wire between us.

The wheels within wheels kept turning. A gay man sprang to his feet and raged against the whole group for being responsible for the persecution of homosexuals. After he'd bashed hell out of his parents for denying him he acknowledged that he'd never felt comfortable within himself about his sexuality. His real rage was at his own ambivalence and this was the first time in his life he'd ever felt safe enough to say that. My heart went out to him.

A lot of rockets were fired and by midnight every single person had worked out either upstairs or in front of the group. One that touched me particularly was a young woman whose father had died in a fire. All she'd ever had of him to bury was a burnt shoe, a bunch of keys and his ring. She had no anger, she said, but wanted to make a symbolic grave out of all the ripped-up phone books. She kissed the truncheon and laid it tenderly on the pile and cried her goodbye to him. Another beautiful young woman had never been able to mourn the death by suicide of her lover or go to his funeral because he was married and his family didn't know about her. She said her goodbyes too.

So much ghastly agony making any troubles I've ever had seem self-indulgent and insignificant by comparison.

The extraordinary thing about these ritual story tellings, these revelations and outpourings, is that they are exactly what tribal societies instinctively provide – the permission and safety to puke it all up. Amazonian Indians, Eskimos, Aborigines, Africans – all have regular occasions with music or dancing, a circle and some kind of rite or magic that allows this release. You can foam at the mouth or roll on the ground in convulsions. You can fall into people's arms for support, weep or holler and nobody thinks it's odd. (I saw the same phenomenon at work once in a popular revivalist church in Nashville, Tennessee.)

What is especially impressive here at this workshop is the tolerance, lack of coercion and absence of hysteria.

The last but one person to share her troubles was a seventy-one-year-old nun – a very surprising impressive woman, with a fund of gentle wisdom and strength. She was worried that she would be inadequate in her new job as Mother Superior to a hospice of very old sisters. She had sat there blinking calmly with pale eyes in her little round face while the chap had blasphemed and raged against the hypocrisy of the Church. 'I agree with him,' she said. 'Everyone in this room is probably a damn sight more loving than most of the pathetic, damaged, so-called religious people who claim to be good and holy. Too much spiritual crap and not enough honesty about natural physical reality,' she went on, astonishingly. 'I only hope I will know enough to be able to serve my old ladies well.'

'Thank God they are getting you,' said Elisabeth. 'They don't know how lucky they are.' Everyone broke into spontaneous applause. Sister Agnes blushed with pleasure.

There was one more person who hadn't spoken: an elderly retired vicar with Parkinson's disease. He had to be painfully helped to his feet and it took an eternity for him to shuffle to the front. In a very weak and tremulous voice he told of the most important and difficult lesson he'd had to learn: to be totally dependent on others after a lifetime of active service as a minister. Having to learn to receive, for a change, instead of giving all the time is hard and humbling but has its valuable place in the scheme of things. Old age and crippling illness both have that lesson to teach, he said, and then he sat down.

Elisabeth believes that euthanasia gets an absolute veto for this reason; you rob the dying person of what may be the most important stage of his growth.

'The windstorms of life put you through the tumbler,' she says. 'It's your choice whether you end up crushed or polished.'

Thursday 13 September

I came late to breakfast this morning and the only vacant seat was next to Conny, the Nazi officer's daughter. We sat in awkward silence for a while then I had an impulse to ask if she would like to try a little healing session together during the afternoon break. She nodded and we both suddenly put our arms around each other. A couple of tears dripped into the cornflakes.

Later when I was out walking by myself in the surrounding woods, I saw a lone figure coming towards me on the path. As it drew nearer I could see it was Helga, the other German woman. 'Hello, I'm from Germany,' she said simply with infinite sadness in her voice.

'Hello, I'm Jewish,' I answered, and words were useless. We held each other and cried a bit, knowing with unspoken certainty that the pain and hate could end here if we wanted it to. I invited her to join Conny and me in our little endeavour to put the world to rights.

So there we were, three middle-aged women sitting in the sun in a private corner of a quiet grassy garden. None of us knew any formula for what we were about to attempt but we sat rather shyly together, eyes closed, facing each other and holding hands. We all knew that something more portentous, more miraculous than mere coincidence had brought us to this moment, so with all the sincerity and genuine true-hearted intensity of which we were capable we tried to send a current of pure love energy round our circle of linked hands first to the left, then to the right, and finally into a thunderous fountain.

It was an experience of incomparable power and rapture – for about twenty minutes we were lifted on great wings and a shower of golden stars rained down on us. Nothing needed to be said, we were like three little kids whose magic wish had been granted, so we went off with our arms around each other to have a cup of tea. The migraine I'd had all week was gone.

All of today's workshop business was Elisabeth talking about death and transition. She speaks with simplicity and certainty, never trying to impose an opinion but drawing you into her vision of the truth, borne out by the documented accounts of many people who have had near-death experiences.

At the moment of death, she says, you pass from the physical realm where you leave the poor old chrysalis. Your butterfly is born and travels towards an incandescent light where those who have loved you and preceded you in death will be waiting. You will be whole again, able to be anywhere with the speed of your thoughts and all knowledge will be yours.

I hope she is right. It is a very comforting view and no less plausible than any other.

She has an extraordinary charisma which springs from her inner peace and courage. She never doubts the miracle-working power of unconditional love or her own gifts. When I've watched her during the course of the last few days, focusing her beam on whoever was on the mat, she never let her intense concentration waver for a second. She is fearless and whole herself so she is confident and able to deal with the homicidal rages or seemingly bottomless chasms of grief that people throw up. Because she is sure it's safe, everybody else feels sure as well and the enfolding circle acts as a cradle – a womb. She says there is a potential mass murderer in every group but if they have the courage to face their own suppressed fear of violence and beat it out in safety on an inanimate object they will never harm a fly.

Throughout the day the compassion and warmth, which until now have been general and encircling, started to become more tactile. People were hugging and embracing and talking together with great affection and openness. We were all each other's healers, surrounded by an amniotic fluid of deep empathy, unconditional love and acceptance. It was a balm and a delight to find oneself able both to give and receive in this atmosphere – miraculous in fact, because it gave a feeling of utter conviction, even to the most cynical amongst us, that there is a dimension that lies beyond the commonplace. An unarguable demonstration that the power of love is invincible and nature is more astonishing than we even dare to dream.

This was the last evening and anyone that wanted to could invite a guest to our final pine-cone ceremony. As dusk came we went outside where a little bonfire had been made. Everyone was carrying a pine cone collected from the woods during the course of the day. We formed a circle (by now about a hundred strong) with arms around each other and sang a few songs. Then one by one, in no prearranged order but like a lovely ballet it flowed so spontaneously, people stepped forward into the firelight and stated what they would like to rid themselves of and leave behind forever – this is embodied in the pine cone which is thrown on the fire. Then they said what they would like to take away with them and stepped back.

People made some beautifully moving and simple declarations. Annie, the nurse, said, 'I want to leave behind "bloody men" and take home my love for my husband.' Her husband had come to be with her and his eyes went all misty. He took her in his arms and they kissed.

The pretty young girl disabled by spina bifida as a baby, who had beaten out a hell of a lot of anger and resentment at her over-protective parents over the last few days, had invited her mum to be her guest, and as she threw away her pine cone she said, 'I want to leave behind self-pity so I can say for the first time in my life, "I love you, Mummy."' And she rushed to hug her mum, who was overcome with happiness.

I said I wanted to leave behind old hatred between people and take home harmony and hope. Then Conny stepped out and said: 'When my parents died I inherited their house in Frankfurt where I now live. In it there is one room that I have never cleared out. It is full of rubbish they left behind although underneath I think there might be some valuable things. Today with Allegra and Helga we made a fountain of golden stars. I am going to throw away the rubbish and take home the stars.' And she threw her pine cone on the fire.

It was an ancient human rite. The fire, the circle, the public declaration, the symbolic discarding and affirmation. When all the pine cones were smoke in the night air there was a little bread and wine followed by dancing and singing. It was very merry and enjoyable and everyone let their hair down in a great cathartic release.

Finally, we all sang 'Wherever Thou goest, I will go' in beautiful improvised harmony. It was the sound of striving and trying and ineffable sweetness. I hear it still.

Friday 14 September

In my suitcase when I got home I found a little drawing of three women in a fertile landscape. On the back it said, 'With love from Conny in memory of a golden fountain.'

I thought of Browning's poem:

> Truth is within ourselves
> . . . and to know
> Rather consists in opening out a way
> Whence the imprisoned splendour may escape.
> > *Part I, Paracelsus Aspires*

3

Those Who Know Have Wings

On the edge of a peaceful Scottish village – the last property before the fields and woods sweep away into the hills, is Bruce MacManaway's home, where he and his wife Patricia have created the Westbank Healing and Teaching Centre, a gushing spring of healing activity and energetic dissemination of ideas. Bruce does not conform to any stereotyped cliché of a witch but a couple of hundred years ago he would undoubtedly have been put to death for his heretical views. There is nothing of the wild-eyed wizard about him, however; he is a tall, practical, reassuring man with military bearing and a direct manner.

A professional soldier for many years, he discovered his healing gifts quite by accident as a young officer in the Second World War. All around him during the French campaign in 1940, men under enemy fire were suffering appalling injuries and there were no proper medical facilities or anaesthetics to help them. Filled with compassion and a terrible feeling of impotence, he laid his hands on the wounded and found to his astonishment that he could alleviate pain, stop bleeding and calm shell-shocked nerves. In the face of considerable scepticism and hostility he had the courage to pursue and develop his skills all through the forties and fifties when healing wasn't fashionable at all. He knew he had stumbled upon something important even though he had no idea how it worked, and felt compelled to follow it up.

In 1959 he was encouraged by Patricia to found Westbank, into which patients began to pour in ever-increasing numbers, enabling him to give up his job as a pigman on a nearby farm and become a full-time healer. He has no formal qualifications but has evolved his own distinctive style based on what he knows works for him. Patricia teaches yoga, grows organic produce and cooks imaginative vegetarian meals for the resident students. Together they have raised three fine sons who have all inherited the healing genes.

I had heard of his reputation from quite a few sources. He has many remarkable cures to his credit in spite of the fact that, as with most alternative practitioners, people usually only come to him as a last resort, after having failed to respond to orthodox treatment. Bruce, in fact, doesn't care for the term 'alternative' and repeatedly asserts that he never seeks to undermine or supplant the medical profession, only to augment it. Anyone can do it, he says, and the ability to receive inspiration can be developed. Revelation and ecstatic vision are not necessarily the preserve of saints and mystics. He believes we all have gifts, some spectacular, some humble. His tireless mission is to further understanding into the nature of healing and to spread confidence in its worth as a complementary therapy. I am predisposed to agree with his claim that healing works regardless of the subject's belief and I wanted to learn some of his specific physical techniques so I joined a group of sixteen would-be healers on a five-day residential course at Strathmiglo. The whole place has a lovely atmosphere and the seminars are held in a large sunny converted barn with Patricia's monster azaleas filling the room with colour.

Every morning began with an optional yoga class taken by Patricia. I was glad to have the opportunity to acquire the basic rudiments. I've learned the hard way that sitting around at healing seminars can make you feel very unhealthy unless you get some exercise. We did forty-five minutes of gentle introductory breathing and relaxation techniques followed by a few postures designed to stretch and coax the body into a state of suppleness and grace. It was enough to make me want to learn more – a lovely way to be nice to your body regardless of age or present state of health. The best thing about yoga is that you can go at your own pace, making things harder or easier according to your capabilities. It is non-competitive, and even bed-ridden and disabled people can derive some benefit from an adapted version.

Bruce talked provocatively about the historical aspects of healing work and the great morass it fell into in early Christian times when an exclusive, professional, all-male priesthood gained control, denying the laity, and especially women, any access, labelling it all as diabolical and zealously trying to root it out. All of this reached its horrific apex during the period of the Inquisition and witch-hunt hysteria, when people were done to death on the merest suspicion of heresy. In England, the witch-craft laws carrying the death penalty were only repealed as recently as 1951! Bruce feels very strongly that orthodox Christianity has a lot to answer for, especially St Paul with his misogyny and his misrepresentation of Christ's message.

'Jesus never set Himself up to be the unique son of God,' says Bruce. 'Only someone in touch with the highest healing power. Why else would He have said "Go and do ye likewise", endorsing forever the value and desirability of lay healers?'

We tried some simple scanning techniques, trying to ascertain whether we could feel a diagnostic or sensing power in our hands. Women are meant to be especially good at this as they can operate more easily at a level of diffuse awareness rather than using the purely focused consciousness associated with masculine thinking, although, of course, plenty of men have this quality too and plenty of women can think in a straight line, so one has to be careful not to generalize on grounds of gender. Certainly diffuse awareness comes easily to me; it must be a survival requirement for mothers. Many times I've found myself stirring the gravy, watching the baby, answering the telephone, wondering what the twins are up to and reading a recipe simultaneously. I know my husband can't do that. He blots out everything but the matter in hand, keeps his eye on the antelope, so to speak. What a pity that over the centuries 'women's intuition' and 'old wives' tales' have been so derided and undervalued.

I could feel a tingling heat in my hands when we were working with partners, and a discernible energy field outside a person's body, but I had no confidence in being able to home in on anything or tell what was wrong or what to do about it. However, after our vegetarian lunch we were shown how to use a pendulum as a tool for dowsing. As Bruce explains it, dowsing is derived from the ancient capability of water divining known in many parts of the world. Practitioners of this art use rods, twigs or pendulums which respond by twitching or rotating and can indicate positive or negative answers to specific questions. There's not a lot of call for water diviners in Britain today, but Bruce, with the help of the British Society of Dowsers, has applied some of the techniques to his healing work. Dowsing, he says, seems to form a bridge for bringing to the conscious understanding of the intellect factors that are known in the subconscious, and is therefore a marvellous help in diagnosis. Contrary to popular belief there's nothing magic about a pendulum; it doesn't actually tell you anything, it doesn't have a mind of its own. What it does is augment and amplify what you already 'know' at a deeper level. You, the healer, are the dowsing instrument. I feel very happy to hear that in so many words, as I've always felt a bit confused about what actually is going on with divination, whether it's tea-leaves or entrails or tarot cards. I suspect it's the same sort of thing at work – your intellect is asking a question and your intuition is supplying the answer; the pendulum is just a visual aid, helping you connect your conscious mind with your unconscious. As with an old-fashioned crystal set, the signal can be quite faint and hard to interpret – a pendulum swinging from your fingers acts like an amplifier and loudspeakers, making the message much clearer.

Of course, a lot of what we call intuition is just a hair's breadth away from imagination and fantasy and it's important to keep our powers of judgement alert. You can't ever trust it completely but you have to be able to follow hunches, have confidence in your judgements and build upon your intuition with more and more experience. It's important to check and double-check all the time.

We borrowed pendulums made from semi-precious stones to practise with. Mine was a piece of rose quartz hanging on a thread. I confess to having felt a certain scepticism about this working for me but I tried it anyway. There are only five answers a pendulum can give. The first thing you do is ask yourself what movement of the pendulum signifies 'yes' for you; then 'no'; 'neutral'; a qualified 'yes'; a qualified 'no'. Every time I tried this I got very clearly differentiated movements! I was really trying not to nudge it round or influence the swing in any way, but it definitely went anti-clockwise for 'yes' and clockwise for 'no'. Perhaps there is a use for it after all. However, when I tried to apply it usefully to diagnostic questions I didn't get very far. The skill lies in asking all the relevant questions.

Bruce asked me to be a volunteer while he demonstrated. Quick as a flash his pendulum whizzed about answering his questions. Did I have trapped nerves? Locked muscles? Stiff bones? Crunched vertebrae? Yes. Yes. Yes. Fifth to sixth thoracic? Yes. Lumbar sacral? Yes. He leaned on my back, cracked and stretched, pummelled and pushed. I could feel it releasing magically. Not a job for an amateur, but whatever he did was superb. I felt at least one inch taller.

After the tea break Bruce had some real live patients who'd consented to being used for teaching purposes and came along to have their treatments done in front of us. The idea was for us to monitor Bruce's diagnoses with our pendulums to see if we picked up the same clues. First a woman who'd recently been in a car crash and suffered whiplash; she had headaches, stiff neck and jaw and attendant depressions. She got some similar treatments to mine, and then Bruce selected certain members of our group (using the pendulum to choose people with sympathetic energies) to do laying on of hands.

Another woman had put her back out. We all formed a great chain to lay on hands, creating, we hoped, a highly magnified beam. She said she could feel enormous comforting heat and quite a lot of pain relief.

The one that specially interested me was a big burly butcher who suffered from terrible pains in his legs and ankles. He'd tried every form of conventional treatment to no avail – no one could find anything wrong with him and I was surprised to hear he'd never even been asked what he did for a living. Bruce is sure that the occupational hazard of continuous heavy lifting has contributed to his condition and caused the rigid congested muscles on either side of the sacral region. He'd been three times already and Bruce had been working on loosening him up. This time he got two volunteers to lay hands on his legs and a third at the top of the spine, then he himself did a deep probing muscle massage using thumbs and elbows to dig in and soften up the tension. I expressed interest in the massage side and got asked to work on the other side of the back. We worked on the man for over an hour – a bit like meat tenderizing, but he certainly felt more supple afterwards. I would be interested to know if he felt a permanent benefit; I felt quite exhausted. It's obviously important to know how to conserve your own strength.

Bruce talked a lot about the spine – the area he focuses on for healing. He uses the term 'levels of awareness' to describe the places along the spinal column which correspond with the chakra system and with the ductless glands of the endocrine system. In his view, everything that happens in the body, whether from a physical or an emotional cause, can be traced to that point on the spine where the nerves emerge from the protective sheath of the spinal column. Congestion and tension, blockages and traps prevent the natural harmonious flow of energy. These blocks are a sign that there is either too much or too little energy input or output at these junctions. He makes an analogy with a bathtub: if there is a blockage in your pipes you won't get enough water flowing through the taps and of course if you can't turn the taps off your bath will overflow all over the place, creating havoc. If you've lost the plug you will be a bottomless pit and no amount of filling will ever be enough.

All this compels us to work constructively on the cause-and-effect cycles within our own bodies. The healer can help by applying deep muscle massage and energy transmission to the corresponding area on the spine that relates to the blocked chakra. Intuition, in this case enhanced by the use of the pendulum (or some other amplifier), guides the healer to the appropriate region and helps in selecting the best form of treatment. Bruce emphasizes that none of the treatment here can be in the least harmful, so even if the patient can't discern an immediate improvement, one has perhaps enabled an orthodox medical practitioner to make further headway.

The spine, he says, is a wonderful diagnostic indicator for the dowser and if one is speaking in terms of cure rather than simple relief, it is the spine, the source of the trouble, that one must treat rather than the area where the pain is manifesting itself (perhaps in a headache or a rheumatic knee).

Bruce described the cycle of damage in layman's language: a nerve gets trapped in the spine for one reason or another, the flow of the bloodstream is hindered, therefore dead cell tissue is not efficiently eliminated or renewed; muscles become hardened or congested, which further grips the nerves, causing more pain, tension, and spasm. These levels of awareness or chakras (he prefers a minimum of jargon and fancy foreign words and I'm sure a large measure of his success is connected with his no-nonsense, reliable, military-man approach) each have their own symbolic language. The illnesses we produce are in each case an appropriate shriek to draw attention to the changes that need to take place.

He also spoke about the contemporary problem of the frustrated flight/fight response and the damage caused by the congestion of adrenalin. At times of stress when the body automatically prepares itself for battle or running away a lot happens in a flash. Blood is withdrawn from the extremities to minimize the loss of blood through injury and to boost supplies to the heart and lungs; a clotting agent is released into the bloodstream, again to minimize bleeding; muscles are primed for strength; pain centres are dulled. What then happens to all this if you are merely fuming in a traffic jam or getting an engaged signal on the phone? You have no way to discharge it other than by domestic violence or shouting at your secretary, so you absorb it into yourself and the tensions build up. They lodge in two prime locations: neck and shoulders or hips and lower back. Hands up anyone who hasn't felt tension in one of those places.

We tried a meditation drawing light and energy up through the levels, to re-charge them, and dispelling tensions and rubbish down through our feet into the earth, which magically transforms waste into nutritious compost. I'm finding the imagery and meditation very much easier than I used to and nearly always get strong visualizations. While working on somebody's spine I saw a powerful field of energy humming and circulating around me. It looked like the ring around the planet Saturn. Helpful images like this make the transmission and channelling part of the process seem natural and obvious.

Throughout the week Patricia provided delicious wholesome food: organic vegetables, red and black currants from the garden and home-made yoghurt. There was also plenty of time off for long walks. Important to keep the temple of the living God in good shape while all these new demands were being made on the spirit.

One evening we joined forces with the regular Monday night meditation group or 'rescue circle'. Bruce with his matter-of-fact, reliable, plausible manner explained its purpose and for someone new to these ideas it sounded barmy and bizarre in the extreme. Lost souls who for one reason or another won't accept that they are dead are wandering around in limbo, he said. Caught up in the trauma of their death they are unable to let go. They need intercession on the part of a sympathetic group to help them on their way. Okay, I'll go along with anything so long as it's not harmful in any way, and the motive here is entirely altruistic.

We sat in a horseshoe formation leaving a space at the north end for our departed chums to join us. We had a candle, a Celtic cross and a symbolic painting of a spiritual pilgrimage to focus our thoughts on. The Celtic cross, explained Bruce, is a beautiful synthesis of pagan and Christian symbolism. It represents in its vertical line the spine of man rooted in the earth and aspiring to the heavens, in its horizontal line the energy, the will, the input of consciousness into the eternal and at its crux, the flower, the lotus, the awareness, the unfolding, the wisdom, a metaphor for mental transformation and the opening up of the psyche. The circle represents the sun, the love of God, benevolence.

Anyway, with all these aids we set off on our mental journeys, Bruce guiding us and our disembodied guests to a place where many people were gathered in an amphitheatre in the presence of a Great Being of Light. I conjured up everything he suggested and sailed off but was never quite asleep. Some people had very powerful reactions. Many felt the presence of the absent friends, many felt they were being approached by spirits who wanted to use them as mediums. I don't think I am medium material but I'd love to have that certainty, one way or the other. I was well aware that the outside world would regard us as insane but actually nothing felt out of place. Hope the poor lost lambs found their way home.

Bruce talked quite a bit about his theories, nay, his knowledge, of reincarnation. I still have enormous problems with that concept although I'm happy to accept that this isn't 'it'. I feel that most ideas about reincarnation are simplistic and banal. My guess is that the reality is outside our present limits of understanding and perception. Different levels of being? A cyclical rather than a linear concept of time? Another universe? Who knows? I'm quite willing to speculate, but a sort of cosmic snakes and ladders where 'I' survive intact and have to come back as another person next time to pay off my karmic debts seems to display a paucity of imagination. I can't believe it's going to be that boring.

By the middle of the week credulity was stretched to the limit and I was never quite sure either that it wasn't a great leg-pull or that Bruce wasn't as mad as a hatter. And yet underneath it all I detect an important lesson for me, and this, I think, is the essence of his teaching. Expansion of awareness, he calls it. Not always needing to have logical answers that fit neatly into what we already know. Being willing to accept different realities, from the realm of imagination and intuition, because they are particularly valid in the healing arts and link directly with ancient, esoteric knowledge. He never gives you a straight answer. There is never, in fact, one answer. He always manages to incorporate everyone's interpretation of a problem (even if they're totally contradictory) as perfectly normal and acceptable.

'Great!' he says emphatically, if anyone offers a point of view, and insists that everybody has some aspect of the ESP gift. He defines ESP not as extrasensory perception, which implies the development of some mysterious paranormal power, but as expanded or extended sensory perception – using what we have but allowing ourselves to be more open, developing new frames of reference, not requiring scientific proof all the time but enabling inspiration to make its own connections. Great steps forward in the history of thought have always come out of our uniquely human capacity to conceive of the possible – to build hypotheses. 'Let's try it, it just might work!' as the hero always says in direst peril when there's nothing to lose.

Colin Wilson put it well. 'Man's consciousness is as powerful as a microscope; it can grasp and analyse experience in a way no animal can achieve. But microscopic vision is narrow vision. We need to develop another kind of consciousness that is the equivalent of the telescope.' He believes that civilization cannot evolve any further until the so-called 'occult' is taken for granted on the same level as atomic energy.

There is nothing of the guru about Bruce. He neither needs nor seeks disciples. He chucks out handfuls of seeds in the hope that some of them will land on fertile soil, always encouraging people to develop their own style. 'I don't give a damn if you believe what I say, there is no dogma. I am merely presenting material for your investigation, techniques for expanding your awareness. Remember we are not doing healing, we are channelling it. We are creating an atmosphere, providing a facility.'

Since healing is the process of 'becoming more whole', as he says, then obviously the more tools you have in your psychic tool box the better. The vital element of training, he stresses, is that we are in a process of growth. If we can develop our sensitivity and awareness we will also develop our healership. 'Please don't think this is *the* way – it's only *a* way,' he says.

His own particular chosen area of focus is the spine and joints for the reasons we went into earlier and also, he asserts, because doctors have been notoriously neglectful of this region. Normal X-rays don't give a picture of trapped nerves or soft tissue in spasm whereas the pendulum, which is amplifying subtle whispers of inner knowing, shows up all sorts of things that the medical profession often doesn't even think to look for. He reminds us again that the skill of this method consists in asking yourself all the possible relevant questions and then fine-tuning your responses. It's really a process of elimination. When a patient comes to him he first dowses for straightforward spinal adjustments, then soft-tissue disturbances (muscles, ligaments, sinews, cartilage), then the organic system (liver, kidneys, etc), food allergies, relationship problems, environmental (is the architectural form of the house harmonious?). A lot of our illnesses, he believes, come from forcing ourselves to live in unsympathetic buildings with shapes not conducive to human well-being. Curves suit us better than straight lines. Do ley-lines (lines of magnetic earth energy, good or bad, positive or negative) run through the house?

The art lies in knowing which questions to ask. Obviously the more possibilities you consider the more you are attuning yourself to the patient's signals both overt and subliminal. Bruce's pendulum is going nineteen to the dozen. He likes the method, he says, because it is so quick, portable and adaptable. Bruce even claims to be able to dowse over a map or ground plan of someone's house to spot the lines of energy, if their ailment appears to be environmental in origin. These magnetic earth currents, he maintains, are as real and as potent as electricity cables or underground streams. The ancients apparently had extensive knowledge of this potent force and placed their sacred sites, temples, standing stones and altars at auspicious intersections accordingly. Many of these have now been insensitively violated, we were told, and the energy flow interrupted by the building of dams, mineshafts, car parks and other such profane monstrosities. This causes the ley-lines to 'go black' and can, in turn, have a very adverse effect on the physical and emotional health of people living in the vicinity . . .

This was all a bit advanced, not to mention weird, and I felt as if I'd just learned to knit – clumsy and slow. But I'm trying hard to keep an open mind.

We were invited to go into the garden to dowse with our pendulums around the area where Bruce said several ley-lines converged on his garden. We were to see how many we could find and report back. If anyone had wanted visual proof of a bunch of English eccentrics in action they should have made a film of us solemnly pacing up and down dangling our little strings or holding our dowsing rods. Probably everyone felt as much of a twit as I did but no one refused to do it, and in fact everyone claimed to feel something.

Bruce is so positive. In this sense he reminds me of Charles Berlitz and his Lost City of Atlantis. He takes you along with him into the realm of the fanciful and you begin to think, 'Well, why not?' There's always the remote possibility that it all makes sense. 'Anyone want to experience a riser?' says Bruce cheerfully, and shows us where an invisible fountain bursts up through the ground in his garden rather like a geyser or an Icelandic hot spring. I couldn't feel anything in the place where he said it was but I thought it was interesting that my first impression of Westbank was of a gushing spring of energy. One wag in our group suggested the site of a riser would be a good spot to have an orgy, but it was a rather chilly Scottish April afternoon so we went back indoors to have a cup of tea instead.

The concept of lines of energy on the earth's surface is something I can accept without any difficulty. I've felt it myself in places like Glastonbury, Dartmoor, Assisi, St Paul's Cathedral and my own house: places where I resonate with sympathetic vibrations and my own energies are amplified by being in a particular spot. It can't be pure accident that so many ancient sacred sites are linked to one another in straight lines along a sort of global grid.

People were picking up forty, fifty, sixty ley-lines in Bruce's garden. I tried hard to do it seriously and got three rather wishy-washy anti-clockwise swings with my bit of rose quartz. I certainly didn't feel any confidence or conviction about it. 'There are three significant bands,' stated Bruce to my astonishment. But he assured all those crestfallen dowsers who had divined lots that there were additional splinters and underground currents that their extra sensitivity had obviously picked up. No one is allowed to feel discouraged.

I developed a bad headache when we were doing that experiment in spite of the fact that Bruce had applied heavy thumb pressure to the back of my neck earlier on to try and relieve the sinus congestion from the tail end of a bad cold. It seemed worse rather than better although, again, he warns everyone that might happen. We then had a chance to work with a partner on diagnosis and treatment. Ken and I chose each other – he was a gentle, elderly widower with a tragic longing to get some kind of message to let him know that his late wife was all right in the spirit world. Some sort of 'proof' that they'd see each other again. I thought that was the main reason why he was here but I also thought he had some fine, sensitive healing skills and might well find a whole new fulfilment in helping others to feel better. I tried to tell him that perhaps this was the very thing his wife would want him to do since his thoughts of her had led him here and would lend him the strength he needed. That in itself was 'proof' of her continued existence and whenever he wanted to think about her, there she would be, encouraging him and helping him. Anyway, that's my philosophy about people dying – you never really lose them because no one can take away what you shared.

We did a scan and dowse and I suddenly felt enormously confident in treating him – the first time that had happened. I just knew what to do: a lengthy deep massage on his shoulders, which released a chronic stiff neck he'd had for ages. He said it was spot on and he was amazed to have the freedom of movement again, which was all very gratifying and confidence-inspiring for me. He worked on my headache, and it gradually dispersed. A pleasurable feeling of being cared for was perhaps the nicest part of all. Once again I was reminded of how important it is to allow oneself to receive.

One day an outside patient came in with a bad itchy skin complaint. Her history was that she'd lived in the same house since she was four years old. Her mother had died, her brother and sister gone to live elsewhere and she'd stayed to look after her elderly disabled father who had Parkinson's disease and an amputated leg. She'd inherited the house and when she'd recently married, her husband had moved in too. They'd extended the house but ever since the time of the marriage she'd experienced a worsening of the rash. Well, I must say I would have looked to find some sort of psychological conflict between looking after an incapacitated old man and enjoying newly married bliss, but the young lady's dermatologist had actually referred her to Bruce. 'Adverse earth radiation,' said Bruce immediately and drew in a black ley-line on the plan of her house. Also he said there was a definite blockage in her spine at that chakra which deals with allergies and skin troubles. She lay on the table and he made some spinal adjustments and got a team of us to lay on hands. The rest of us turned ourselves into a circle of healing energy to enfold her and before she left she was given a massive iron bar to 'pin' the ley-line in her house. She was to ring up that evening and Bruce would dowse for the exact place to put it within a couple of millimetres.

After she'd gone he demonstrated how to use the pendulum and ask all the necessary questions ranging from the physical to the environmental. He's found that sometimes when a food allergy has been suspected, he has been able to pick up the fact that rather than the foodstuff itself being the cause of the trouble, the allergy is due to the preparation or the packaging material instead. Very useful for someone to know, for instance, that they can eat virtually anything so long as it's not wrapped in plastic.

As the sun went down and the evening session ended a few of us walked to the top of East Lomond. It is an old Druid site and Roman fortification with powerful ley-lines allegedly running straight down to Bruce's garden – indeed in through his bedroom window. It was very cold up there, but beautiful, with views all over the surrounding countryside right to the coast and an intensely red globe of a sun hanging like a ripe tomato in the sky. When I tried to dowse for the ley-lines, I'm sorry to say, my pendulum just blew about in the wind.

Bruce began a talk on mediumship one morning with remarks about the 'so-called dead' which really set the tone for the whole discussion. According to him they are just beings who have been liberated from the restrictions of the body and live in the wider consciousness with a wider range of options open to them. The trouble is, we have largely lost confidence in setting up communications with them, unlike, say, the Japanese or the Aborigines who have a very jolly relationship with their ancestors and regularly consult them on matters of importance.

This present-day sorry state of affairs all came about because of the Christian Church's rabid witch-hunting paranoia and Bruce makes the analogy fairly graphic by saying, 'What if an Inquisition were set up to root out and execute all telephone engineers? You'd still have an excellent telephone system left but no one would know how to operate it.' Obviously, as with any skill, some people are better communicators than others. If you don't happen to be brilliant at it yourself, he says, don't be ashamed to consult a professional medium. After all, if you didn't have a private phone in your house you wouldn't shun a public call box!

He gave some tips on what to do if you decide to consult a medium. For example, don't give your real name, especially if you're well known; don't fall for leading questions, make them work for the answers rather than blurting out everything and declaring your recognition too soon; try to get some validation – answers to questions of which only you would know the significance, for example. He warned that people may well try to put you off, claiming that it's dangerous or heretical. Disregard all their faulty arguments against communicating. 'After all, if God didn't want us to do it, why did Jesus teach it? The beginning of the development of mediumship is to open yourself to the possibility.'

Perhaps the fact that I'm only very reluctantly allowing the possibility here is the reason why I'm not very gifted in this department. I am really trying to be open-minded but I'm also wary of being too gullible. This has always been an orchard of ripe pickings for unscrupulous frauds and confidence tricksters preying on the vulnerable and lonely. Perhaps that's at the root of my resistance. Ultimately one can only go by 'gut feeling', and 'gut feeling', after all, is an ESP faculty.

Bruce sat inscrutably in his chair, looking dependable and calm, kindly and fatherly, wearing a T-shirt that day that bore the inscription, 'Life is Too Short to Waste Time Hurrying'. He is a great yea-sayer, full of energy and enthusiasm. He busily wove a net big enough to encompass any illogical inconsistency, saying that whatever happened would be perfectly in order and adding that you must allow a wide margin for human error and imperfection, spiritual con men, and the reluctance of some spirits (mainly departed husbands!) to get in touch with their loved ones.

Just because you don't understand what's happening doesn't of course prove that it can't happen. After all, you can watch television or drive a car without understanding the first thing about electronics or mechanics. The very thing we are trying to do with our expanded awareness is to allow the possibility for any ESP skill to manifest itself. Everyone has some gifts, but you don't necessarily have them all. Bruce quotes St Paul's first letter to the Corinthians – Chapter 12:14 – concerning spiritual gifts: 'But the manifestation of the Spirit is given to every man to profit withal.' And goes on to enumerate these gifts: to one is given the word of wisdom; to another the word of knowledge; to another faith; to another the gifts of healing; to another the working of miracles; to another prophecy; to another discerning of spirits; to another divers kinds of tongues; to another the interpretation of tongues. 'If the whole body were an eye, where were the hearing?'

Open yourself, is the essence of Bruce's teaching, and see where you are most gifted. Don't narrow your options by denying these weird and wonderful magic happenings.

I asked him, since he was so convinced of the possibility of communication with guides and benevolent spirits, whether he also believed in the existence of evil spirits and demonic possession. 'Definitely!' he answered, unequivocally. 'You can be mugged in the spirit world just as well as in this one. Evil exists right the way up the evolutionary scale.'

In most parts of the world the dominant theory of both physical and mental sickness has historically been one of possession by spirits or demons. I can't quite see them as outside entities as Bruce does, but I can accept the metaphor. Perhaps we all have our own demons: the powerful, fiery, forbidden side of our natures. The ruling passions when not allowed adequate self-expression or kept sufficiently under control sneak up and devour us. The spiritual muggers! Christianity calls this the Devil, psychoanalysis the id. Priests, psychiatrists and witchdoctors are in business to liberate us from their grasp but eventually we must learn to master them for ourselves.

There is a wide spectrum of practitioners, from bone-rattling sorcerers to exalted Sufi mystics, to whom we can turn for guidance in these matters. They are the ones to give us safe passage on a dangerous journey, whether it be a quiet interior meditation or the space to freak out in safety – knowing there are boundaries to protect you and arms to hold you if you fall. It seems a good idea; all sorts of psychic stresses and culturally unacceptable behaviour or ideas can be given expression in the blameless state of ecstasy until you've literally 'got it out of your system'. I see possession as a reaction to individual conflict and the freak-out as a useful psychological defence.

The first time I was ever really aware of the therapeutic properties of mass ecstasy was a couple of years ago when I stayed a few days with the Reverend Jimmie Snow and his wife Dottie in Nashville, Tennessee. What I saw there fits well into the framework of all I have learned subsequently.

Dottie Snow was there to meet me at the bus depot – I had to arrive in Nashville by Greyhound Bus; it was part of the mythology. Dottie is a gorgeous Nashville doll with a cascading blonde wig like Dolly Parton, and a perfect figure ('I may be the only Bible some of these people will ever read,' she explains). She swept me up in an extravagant welcome and embraced me with open arms. That first night was the only night of the week when the Grand Old Opry Show was on. You can't come to Nashville and not see it – it is the Mecca of country-and-western music lovers from all over the world. Dottie and her family have been in the entertainment business all their lives so she took me straight backstage where she knew everyone from the doorman to the stars and we watched the show from the wings. It's a great hootin' and hollerin' style of popular culture, raucous and sentimental by turns, and it all helped me to set what followed in its rightful context.

I drove to the church, the Evangel Temple, with Dottie next

morning. The congregation is mostly conservative, mostly white but by no means all, of every age from a one-week-old baby to ancient grannies. The place filled up fast and on came the band, several guitars, a banjo, piano, organ, and a large choir including Dottie looking like an angel in a long robe. The Rev. Jimmie Snow seized the microphone and got things rolling with a rousing gospel song. Everyone knew all the songs and joined in with hand clapping and singing. His young curate led some of the numbers – beginning by saying, 'I used to be a heroin addict, now I'm a Jesus junkie. Praise the Lord!' The music went on for an hour. 'How many of you people want to hear some good old-fashioned Holy Ghost organ music?' yelled the Rev. 'Come on, smoke it boy!'

The organist was quite a virtuoso and his wife came up and fanned the keyboard afterwards to cool it down. 'How about that! C'mon you all, let's hear it for God. Give Him a big hand now.' Then Brother Snow began his sermon. He had a bit of trouble with his neck mike to start with but was soon producing a suitable volume. He is a very energetic preacher, stalking the aisles, orchestrating his crescendos, choosing his words effectively. His theme was a verse from the Bible which states something to the effect that 'Happy is the man whose sins shall not be charged against him.' He spoke for over an hour, exhorting us to let Jesus take the load off us. The only way to get to heaven, he said, is to unburden your sins on Jesus – doesn't matter what you've done. He finished off in quite a lather, his shirt soaked with sweat, his pale blue synthetic ultra-suede jacket long since removed. He jumped up and down as if he were on a pogo stick on the stage yelling, 'I been set free by the blood of the Lamb. There are no sins charged to my account. Jesus has put them on His American Express card and He has NO CREDIT LIMIT.' Plenty of 'Hallelujahs!' and 'Praise Gods!'

People certainly had a good time. It was a great show with plenty of audience participation. The Rev. has also been in the entertainment business all his life. His father is Hank Snow, the country-and-western singer. Until he was twenty-two, Jimmie was a singer himself – making plenty of money, singing and travelling with Elvis Presley and others. He was into bad company and bad habits, drugs, booze and women. 'I've woken up in every motel in this town,' he told me. But he saw the light when he was twenty-two, became converted, started preaching and has been at it ever since. The entertainment business and the religion business have superficially got a lot in common here in the Bible Belt and I confess that to my less flamboyant English taste the service was somewhat off-putting, but it's easy to mock the rather more ludicrous elements and fail to perceive what is really happening. The faith, hope and love presented in this exciting high-voltage form are appropriate to the terms of reference of the community, liberating the congregation from the confines of everyday cares and rational thought, providing a socially sanctioned cathartic release – a safe healing space.

Everyone went home for a rest, but Jimmie stayed on at the church to spend a couple of hours working on his sermon for the evening service. During a revival they have two services a day for the whole week. Each one this week was packed. At 7 pm Dottie and I drove over. The service started off the same as before with people singing and clapping. Jimmie was doing nothing special to whip them up but gradually the room just seemed to fill up with an enormous energy force. One by one, people had tears rolling down their cheeks, people standing next to one another reached out and held each other. Arms were uplifted in praise. Some people fainted clean away and others sat beside them with joyous faces, holding and rocking them. Middle-aged men comforted each other's tears. Little children embraced and lifted their arms and asked for Jesus to come to them. People sang and danced and jumped and cried and the music played on. Whatever it was in that room was very powerful and people had made the connection with it – the universal life force? Even a naturally reserved and sceptical British onlooker couldn't fail to feel the power. It wasn't hysteria, it was love and faith and the ability to let go. Jimmie never even tried to preach his sermon. He could see what was happening and he just let it roll.

I saw the same thing happen once at a little praise meeting for the God, Krishna, in Kathmandu. I was taken by a friend who had chosen the Hindu path to enlightenment. They had flower offerings, incense and music and kept up a continuous repetitive chanting. They swooned with adoration and were overcome with transcendental joy.

Whatever the cultural context it seems valuable to be able to release in this fashion. To find a way of relinquishing the self and be willing to let the tide of ecstasy sweep you up.

Now in Nashville, the rapture gradually died down and people composed themselves a bit – stood about talking with their arms around each other and marvelled at how happy and comforted they felt. One woman I talked to afterwards told me that seven years ago her daughter and son-in-law had been having marital problems. The daughter left him and in a fit of jealous madness, he and a buddy kidnapped her back again, hijacked a plane and were stormed by the FBI when they tried to land for refuelling. The guy shot both himself and his wife. They left a three-year-old daughter whom this woman and her husband had adopted. She had a hard time coming to terms with the horrible tragedy and tried going to her old church for comfort but everything seemed cold and meaningless until a friend brought her here to the Evangel Temple and the warmth and strength she has received from the place have healed her to the point where she can cope with life again. Prayer undoubtedly has enormous power. But so has meditation. So has voodoo. I suspect that they are all the same thing – mind power – called by different names and tailored to suit different temperaments and mythologies. Jung uncovered a deep connecting network of universal symbolism that he called 'archetypes' in his explorations of the mind. A sort of inner knowing, a deep organizing system by which we attempt to give meaning to the unexplainable. We thrash about for a framework to fit it into, and have come up with many possible answers. The Rev. Jimmie Snow's church has a good thing going here; I just resent being told it's the only way.

Later on back at his home, I asked Jimmie Snow whether he wasn't worried about the vulnerability and exploitability of the people in his care – it wasn't long since the mass suicide in Guyana of the Rev. Jim Jones's followers had shocked the world. He said the difference between himself and someone like Jim Jones was that while he remained a humble medium for the spirit, Jim Jones assumed the mantle – the power made him drunk and he started to believe he was God, the spirit incarnate. But, yes – people are vulnerable when they first come into the fold. They are very needy and all they have is an intimation, an emotional glimpse, until they've had time to give their faith substance.

I found him to be a genuinely sincere man, a good psychologist, an intelligent questioning thinker and a hard honest worker. His showmanship is part of him and the fact that he uses it as a tool should not fog the issue. He gave me a signed copy of his autobiography, which tells the story of his change from a life of sin to a life for God.

Before I left, Dottie took me out shopping: a surreal experience. They don't have high-street-type shops at all here. Nashville is strung out along identical freeways bordered by petrol stations and fast-food chains. All shopping takes place in vast space stations, air-conditioned indoor piazzas surrounded by mammoth car parks. Nobody seems to go outside, ever, and living takes place in a completely synthetic environment. Dottie runs from her air-conditioned house where the curtains are always drawn and the blinds pulled down, to her air-conditioned car with her sunglasses on, to the air-conditioned shopping precinct with the muzak playing. If the time ever comes to vacate this planet, the Snows would be good people to send off into the stratosphere – they wouldn't miss the earth at all. They even have plastic flowers in the flowerbed outside their front door and plastic waterlilies in their little fountain. They hardly ever eat real food: they drink diet Cokes and instant iced tea. They use 'creamer' in their coffee and 'spread' on their bread and pick up junk food from a take-away when they're hungry. They never have fresh fruit in the house but eat bowls of Baskin-Robbins ice cream or pies warmed up in the microwave. All Dottie's clothes are made of polyester, as are the sheets on their beds, and they have arrangements of artificial flowers in the lounge and dining-room. Their television is projected on to a giant screen that dominates the den and they never turn it off. The teenage boys sleep with the radio playing softly all night. The things I would pine for in outer space, they have already learned to live without.

The shops are abundantly stocked and dream-like. Nobody pays with money – everyone uses credit cards. Dottie took me to the wig shop where she buys her artificial hair. 'I never go out in my real hair any more, a wig is so much more convenient,' she says. I bought a curly mane of strawberry blonde and resolved to enter as fully as I could into the spirit of the place when I went to church for the last time that evening.

Brother Snow was determined to preach the sermon that he'd had prepared since Sunday. The congregation were pretty tired as this revival had been going on all week, so it gave Jimmie the chance to talk to a quiet receptive audience. It was a good sermon, well researched and well structured, about the prophecies in the Bible and how often they've turned out to be true. He is a pretty good Bible scholar and I enjoyed his open, down-home, warm-hearted, style. It is relevant to his congregation, simple, direct, and sincere. Even though, to me, the environment was as foreign as Africa, the point is that the gaudy packaging doesn't diminish our shared human needs and sincere aspirations to find meaning in life.

He finished off by asking if there was anyone in the congregation who would like him to pray for them. I put my hand up – partly because I knew it would please him and Dottie to know that I felt strongly about something that means so much to them, but largely because I feel that they really do have a communion with the unknown quantity that they call God and understand the nature of the healing power of love.

They were ecstatic with joy to think that I had made a commitment. They wept and held me and prayed. But I had to be honest, although I valued the warmth and energy of their prayers. I'm not prepared to be limited to any one system of faith.

'If you have doubts, just open your heart and ask God to prove to you that he's real,' begged Dottie. 'Just try it,' she implored.

'Make that leap of faith, and you'll see that it's true.' Their ardour was touching but I can't accept that you have to follow a leader in order to be a seeker. They are convinced I'll come round so we left it at that.

Now, here in Scotland, a million miles away from Nashville, we had come on to the next stage in our endeavours to push out the frontiers of experience. In the afternoon, our group joined forces with another that meets here regularly every Wednesday to do an 'absent healing' meditation. Unlike the Rescue Circle which is for helping lost souls in limbo, this is for the living who are sick or injured and might benefit from the combined energy projection and healing intentions of a group of people who are focusing their beam on a specific task. As Bruce reminds us, a group is always effectively more than the sum of its parts.

We began by sitting quietly and silently invoking the assistance of any 'guides' or spirits who might be listening. 'You invite them in to share your energy,' suggested Bruce. 'They need us as much as we need them in order to accomplish concrete deeds.' I must admit I have been a bit puzzled by the concept of 'guides'. I asked him, 'How will you know when you have one? Or when? How do they make themselves known?'

'They are always there,' he replied. 'When the time comes that you need some kind of proof, you will know for sure.' He is a sane and sensible man. My immediate sceptical response, my conditioned reflex of discomfort and cynicism, I felt to be unworthy and inappropriate in a context of adventure and discovery. So I resolved to suspend my disbelief and expand my awareness to see if I could sense another facet to my 'knowing', a booster system to my intuition. If it's possible to have guides, beings with a greater knowledge than yours, on your side, what a bonus! And how stupid to disallow it before you start.

This was a very long, deep visualization and meditation led by Bruce, using the visual aid of his painting as a landscape for our thoughts. We were to encourage our subconscious (or whatever that part of the mind is that can take off and go travelling) to link up on a higher level to the power source – a sort of cosmic national grid. Into our circle of care we were to try and incorporate the people whose names he read out and cocoon them in a charge of healing energy.

I flew off quite quickly and easily and as Bruce said each name, I pictured in my mind's eye the person bringing up a chair and joining our gathering, connected to a column of white light in our midst by an umbilical cord made of a rainbow. Now where did that come from? I know I 'thought it up' but there seemed to be more to it than that. It was 'of me', but somehow of a bigger me than I usually use. I felt very uncomfortable, with a dry throat and mouth. My face became very flushed and hot although the room was at a normal temperature. And my hands that were quietly relaxed in my lap began to tingle furiously, almost as if they were in contact with an electric vibrator.

Quite often, when I'm trying to meditate, I see a huge sunflower that fills the whole screen. It appeared again now but for the first time I saw a shadowy figure in front of it, just momentarily. A strong impression of the outline of a person in silhouette at the corner of my mind. When I tried to focus on it more clearly, it slipped out of range like a dream upon waking. I didn't give it much thought but hoped it would return again with more clarity. I confess I was intrigued and excited. If an identifiable, perceivable guide can amplify an inner voice for me or provide a link with another reality (maybe the two things are one and the same?), I want to be listening. I thought about which guides I would ideally choose if I had a say in the matter: my dad? Albert Schweitzer? My old piano teacher, Greta Cohn? But the shape didn't reveal itself.

Now comes the question of delusion, fantasy and imagination. Just because I want to see something, am I kidding myself? How will I know if it's real? How indeed! How could you ever know if romantic love is real? It seems real enough when you're feeling it. The power it gives you is real, the strength, the happiness, all real. So who can say it's an illusion? Is God real? Is hope real? Does belief create the fact? You'll never know in the accepted rational sense, not in a way you could prove to anyone else. I don't honestly think it matters. If it enables you, empowers you, amplifies you, then it's a potent force.

William James, the philosopher, once said, 'Our normal waking consciousness . . . is but one type of consciousness, whilst all around it, parted from it by the filmiest of screens, there lie potential forms of consciousness entirely different.' How can we accept that the trivial reality of everyday preoccupations is all there is? In the Tibetan world view, the dividing line between the real and the imaginary is very soft focus. All that can be imagined is as real as all that exists. They do not distinguish between natural and supernatural. Miracles are merely the clever handling of little-known laws and forces.

Later on, in the same state of altered consciousness, I saw the profile, in a lightning-quick, subliminal flash which I couldn't recapture, of a beautiful woman with very long reddish-gold hair. The instant I came out of the meditation, a story came rushing into my mind, a story I remember my mother telling me when I was little. I know at the time I was moved by the tragedy and romance of it and it certainly would have impressed itself deeply on my child's mind, but I have not consciously recalled it for thirty years or more. My mother's Auntie Violet, my grandmother's younger sister, was a ravishing beauty renowned for her Titian hair. In the First World War she became a nurse and was much loved for her caring gentleness and beauty by the wounded men she looked after. She was serving on a hospital ship transporting casualties when it was torpedoed. She was hit by falling debris and flung unconscious into the icy water. A soldier who had lost both his arms in the fighting saw her going down for the third time and valiantly tried to keep her afloat by grabbing her golden hair in his teeth, but they both drowned.

Auntie Violet is part of me, I carry her genes in my body which connect me to her. Her story is part of my mythology, my racial memory. Why shouldn't she appear in my dreams and meditations? Why shouldn't I be able to draw on her strength and healing skills? I think I feel happier with this concept of a 'guide' rather than with the idea of an actual separate being, a symbolic rather than a literal guide. I have quite a gut resistance to the thought of dead people still floating about intact, but believing that it's 'only in the mind' doesn't seem to diminish the phenomenon at all. We need to maintain good communications with ourselves, between the conscious and the subconscious, between the two hemispheres of the brain, and with the unseen forces whatever they may be.

Your mind can travel through infinite and eternal spaces to the deepest core of your genetic inheritance as a human being. Just because your relations have gone to live in 'another country' it doesn't mean you can never contact them again. You can build a bridge, a ship, a magic carpet.

Although there was no whooping and hollering, no ecstatic or exhibitionist trance state in our sober Scottish ritual, everyone was miles away in their minds, 'visualizing'. Someone felt physically assaulted by the strength of a spirit trying to enter him, someone felt nudged and jostled, someone saw groups of people in circles like flower petals interlocking as far as the eye could see, and symbolic expressions of travelling, especially of ascent, kept on recurring: a boat; a ladder; a vine; a rainbow; a plume of smoke; a sunbeam. Vehicles, rites of passage to the unknown – enabling us to transcend and rise above the clay feet of the human condition.

In shamanic tradition, the same means are employed to ensure the ascent of a dead man's soul. It's as if we have always been looking at the Grand Canyon through a crack in the fence and at last realize that we must raise ourselves high enough to look over the top at the whole scene. All over the world the same magical power of flight is credited to sorcerers and medicine men: changing into birds, riding on broomsticks, levitating, astral travelling. 'Among all things that fly, the mind is the swiftest,' says an American Indian proverb. 'Those who know have wings.'

We have a deep collective nostalgia for the riches that have been stored in a vault for safekeeping all through the ascendancy of the Age of Reason. Stored in 'women's intuition' and 'old wives' tales' and in the minds of mystics and dreamers.

Our little group of absent healers was like a flock of great heavy flightless birds flapping stunted wings like crazy in an effort to take to the air. We should learn a salutary lesson from earthbound ostriches. They have spent so long keeping their feet

84

on the ground and their heads in the sand that they have lost the power of flight forever. Whereas the bumblebee continues to fly despite the fact that science has proved it aerodynamically impossible. I think we might have a second chance; let's not waste it.

It's exciting to recognize the connecting threads between all the methods I've so far sampled to free the mind from the bonds of the intellect and allow it to soar. Linking the Rev. Snow's Evangel Temple, Elisabeth Kübler-Ross's Life, Death and Transition workshop, Andrew Watson's Healing Intensive with the exorcism of devils and the need for ritual, it's interesting to see how wide a range of behaviour is permitted in the healing space and it seems that the function of the healer is to help create that space wherein dynamic change can occur.

Rituals, sometimes bizarre, sometimes beautiful, are a powerful aid to the transformational process. They invoke the altered state. Incense, Palestrina, and the holy sacrament is one way; a bonfire, drums and a head-dress of eagle feathers is another – awakening the power, releasing the feelings, affirming the faith, transcending the ego.

'The use of cultural myth received from the collective tradition,' is how anthropologist Claude Lévi-Strauss describes shamanic healing. He believes that underlying all cultural systems there is a structural similarity and an innate universal consistency. And that these systems, like languages, no matter how different they might superficially seem, will always translate from one to the other because the concepts are interchangeable.

Warring over belief systems is as stupid as warring over languages would be. They're all as good as each other, and although some may be more refined than others, they all serve the same purpose and are basically trying to express the same quest with varying degrees of eloquence: the quest for a healing space.

It would be comical if it wasn't so ghastly – two thousand years of religious wars, of murder, hatred and persecution, of subjugation and domination in the name of 'truth' – the blind men describing the elephant in the Sufi tale. Who dares to lay down the rules and say that only they know the nature of God?

Yesterday, inquisitors were burning witches. Today Hindus and Sikhs cut each other's throats, Muslims and Jews gun each other down, Catholics and Protestants blow each other up, a South African church doesn't accept black worshippers, Christian missionaries disrupt and obliterate the beliefs of tribal societies. Everyone busily imposing, crushing, limiting, denying. Surely only a recognition of the interconnectedness of all these sincere attempts to make sense of our existence will bring peace and harmony to our planet. Our spirituality is our 'healing space', helping us to be the very best that we can be, mind, body and spirit. Bringing the magnifying glass in line with the sun, bringing wholeness to us by any method that works – that is surely the only criterion. It is the underlying intention that counts. Jesus said, 'The Kingdom of Heaven is within you' and taught that our bodies are 'the temple of the living God'. We all have intimations of this and are continually trying to taste the divine nectar, hear the divine melody, see the divine light, find oneness in one way or another.

As Bruce says, 'We lost sight of wholeness many centuries ago when religion and medicine separated.' He is such a refreshing, blunt enthusiast and understands, with a military strategist's cunning, the value of many small cadres infiltrating the barricades. The essence of his teaching about healing is, 'Accept the challenge, get out and do it, don't be afraid.' He emphasizes that Jesus Himself did not form a church or a monolith: 'He formed little self-contained blobs, the most effective form of military defence. And don't forget, you are not in isolation. When in difficulties, send for reinforcements. If you give yourself to things of the spirit, you will get help from the spirit.'

He had told us earlier that our potential abilities were all different, and now a lot of us wanted him to tell us individually what he thought these might be. So, using his pendulum, and making the strong proviso that these talents are only to be pursued when you feel ready – there is no compulsion to follow them unless you wish to – he went round the group dowsing for 'gifts'. I was impressed by his sensitive and intuitive understanding of how much people were ready to hear according to their own inclinations.

To one woman, a good person but a compulsive chatterbox, he said that everything would respond to her hands: animals, plants, the earth, people; but he advised against counselling! To another, a shy, elderly widow, he suggested teaching, dowsing and counselling but warned her not to do too much with her hands. 'People will suck the guts out of you.' To an unconfident young man, the opinion that his vocation lay with healing animals. To a dreamy old man that he had an aptitude for mediumship and working through a guide. To me he said, 'Hands! Very strongly. And dowsing with the pendulum. Your abilities are more practical than mental and there's not much aptitude for communicating with the spirit world. As yet!' he added as an afterthought. He qualified everything by saying none of this is absolute of course, especially the negative predictions, and that no matter where you start you quickly travel into other unexpected dimensions.

'As a diagnostician, recognize and register the physical and the non-physical so that you are constantly aware of your own state of health and well-being,' he reminded us wisely, hinting that there are some blind leading the blind around, who would be well advised to monitor the order in their own houses. 'Just allow yourself to be and resonate with the energy.' He also encouraged us to work in groups. 'Energy is not just an amorphous mass,' he said. 'It is generated at specific frequencies. We are the transformers and work well in a group covering a wide range of frequencies. The pooled resources benefit everyone.' He echoed my little revelation on the top of Brentor on Dartmoor when he reiterated Jesus's statement, 'When two or three are gathered together . . .'

Bruce also recommended getting a training in some specific technique such as massage and a rudimentary knowledge of anatomy to augment our gifts of the spirit. He warned us to be steadfast in the face of opposition, not to allow ourselves to be limited by doctors, priests, or trade unions who all have a vested interest in keeping lay people away from healing.

'Yes, it's dangerous. If you are too easily put off and frightened, don't get involved,' he said bluntly. 'Yes, you will be subjected to psychic attack. Yes, some of you may even be killed. So what? Assess the risk. Some things are worth dying for.'

We came on to the interesting topic of personal protection – of psychic self-defence. Since power is of itself neutral, it can, of course, be harnessed for good or evil, to heal or harm, to cure or curse. All over the world people have invented charms and jujus to ward off the evil eye. Bruce showed us how to make a pattern of pentagons to represent visually the idea of a protection against psychic draining. I thought that was all a bit fiddly and hocus-pocus but I liked the concept of 'the mirror of light': If you think you are the victim of black magic or if you are being bombarded by evil vibes you can picture your tormentor encircled by a cylinder of mirror glass so that all the malevolence is reflected straight back at him. I love it! So simple, like seven-league boots or a cloak of darkness. SHAZAM!

Bruce cautioned against trying to protect ourselves too much, however, implying it would be like trying to make love in a suit of armour. 'You want a flow of energy,' he said. I am constantly delighted by the human capacity for metaphor. Our minds have a natural facility to invent and use symbols. If illness can be seen as a metaphor for disharmony in the body, we can use symbols and rituals to help realign ourselves.

Finally Bruce taught us a little closing sequence to use after a healing or meditation session. It wouldn't do, he said, to go around too wide open in normal everyday life, so this gently draws in your antennae. On each chakra, each gateway, you draw an imaginary cross within a circle, starting at the crown and ending at the base chakra. We are back again with ancient universal symbols from the collective unconscious. The circle signifying wholeness, the cross standing for the body and soul of man. You finish with crossed ankles and folded hands then breathe in seven bands of golden light through your feet, up your spine and out through the top of your head. Spread these bands of light out into a globe that encloses you and seal it with a seven-fold spiral.

The week at Westbank made me think a lot about the centuries of repression and persecution suffered by anyone, especially women, who dared to express or develop their natural God-given gifts of the spirit. The obscene frenzy of the witch-hunt craze and the general derision, ridicule or fear that even today still largely prevails whenever the 'occult' is the subject of discussion. It made me want to find out more about the history of the subject and led to a strange experience of sweet inner knowing that gave me much pleasure and further clarified my understanding of this 'guide' concept.

When my father died eight years ago I had some experiences of closeness with his spirit. The most striking was shortly after his death when I was still pretty stunned with misery and longing for some word of comfort. I was lying in bed, unable to sleep, my mind in a turmoil, when into the midst of my consciousness came these words: 'You can't stop the birds of sorrow from fluttering around your head but you can prevent them from making nests in your hair! God bless you, Lali.' It was his voice in my mind's ear. I felt like someone had drawn a blanket round my shoulders when I was cold, and I fell asleep smiling. Since then I have often felt his benevolent presence within and around me – again those magic words – enabling and empowering me, making me believe that you never really lose someone when they die because they stay in your mind and you can think about them whenever you want.

Six years later when my mother died, I inherited the only material thing he ever cared about, his books – hundreds of them. We built some shelves in a sunny room and this is where I sit and write with a little crystal that hangs in the window, sometimes mischievous, sometimes mystical, dazzling me with its many-faceted representations of the nature of light. There were so many books that I had no idea what was there, we had just sorted them roughly into categories. Suddenly I realized there was a whole shelf of relevant books on the history of sorcery, witchcraft, psychic phenomena, and comparative religious philosophy. They sort of loomed out at me; one even fell off the shelf and a bookmark with some notes scribbled on it in his handwriting fluttered out. I recalled my father's tender laughing face so clearly and had the oddest sensation of the shadow I'd perceived in the corner of my meditation during the absent healing at Westbank beginning to fill out into his shape. The memory of a smell, warm and male, barely suggested itself, just out of reach, and was gone as I thought of him. With a jolt the insight came to me:

'You were here all along,' I said out loud and the sound of my own voice in the empty room surprised me. Of course, you are my guide. You always have been. You and your beloved books and your lifelong interests are an inseparable part of me, helping me to grow, enriching me. I am you and you are me, my companion on this journey to the interior, to an intuitive reality that doesn't need 'proof'. I looked out of the window and my eyes brimmed. Against the background of acacia trees in my garden I saw a Cheshire-cat image of him beaming with pleasure as I made this leap of understanding. The gift of love that he gave is my greatest strength and as my 'guide' he will always stand at the corner of my mind.

I know many people 'see' and 'hear' spirits with whom they have no kinship tie or even any prior conscious awareness. Perhaps they are more advanced than I am but this, to me, at my stage of readiness, is an acceptable way of making sense of the spirit phenomenon. If so many people claim to have communications with 'discarnates' as Bruce calls them, they can't all be liars or frauds. I'm not necessarily looking for a rational explanation but what I suspect is happening with me is an imaginative projection from inside. Young children often have imaginary friends with whom they play quite unselfconsciously until we tell them to stop being silly. Like our sub-personalities and mythical archetypes, they are characters from our unconscious mind – bit players in our mental theatre, ancestral voices that prompt from the wings. Like the moose and the black monk of my daydreams, spirit guides are within me – part of me and yet apart. I can invent them, conjure them, confront them and ask for advice or insights. Like those umbilical rainbows in the absent healing, they are 'of me' but somehow of a bigger me than I usually draw on, real in another dimension like shamanic flight.

Trying to prove the veracity in scientific terms is a pointless exercise that diminishes the poetry and dismantles the butterfly. 'Those who know have wings.'

The moment I returned from Scotland, I went to see my mother's eighty-year-old sister to ask her if there were any photos in existence of her Auntie Violet so I could see what she looked like. She rummaged in a trunk and found one. It was a profile of a beautiful woman with long fair hair. To my knowledge I had never seen it before in my life but it was the very self-same image that had flashed on my mental slide projector and uncovered the hidden memory of my drowned heroine.

4

The Doctor Who Resides Within

One day in a burst of extravagance I rang Ali, a Kikuyu friend in Nairobi, to ask him if he knew any good healers in Kenya. I told him of my interest in healing, holding forth about my views on disease as a manifestation of conflict and being out of harmony with nature. I mentioned that I was particularly interested in the connections and parallels between the ancient shamanic traditions of indigenous African healing practices and the resurgence of spiritual and other 'alternative' healing practices currently enjoying a revival in the West. I hinted at how much I wanted to look at different cultural manifestations of the healing encounter to see what they have in common.

He said what I hoped he'd say: 'Why don't you come to Kenya and see for yourself one of our native doctors at work?' He brushed aside any complications and difficulties with the assurance 'No problem! Just come and we will arrange everything.'

Just come! How would I ever be able to afford it? I went to see the manager of Kenya Airways and with great panache they generously and imaginatively agreed to sponsor my trip in the hope that it might help to further international understanding of the subject. So fortune was on my side, and in an electric air of anticipation, I packed my bags and went.

My plan was to locate a suitable practitioner with Ali's help and ask if he or she would let me be a sort of apprentice – learning, watching, helping, exchanging ideas. It wasn't to be quite as straightforward as that. 'No problem!' That marvellous ubiquitous African phrase is the curse that taunts all achievement-orientated foreigners who challenge the rhythm of life on that mighty continent.

People say it to cheer you up when things are about as chaotic as they can be. When your plans have all collapsed or nobody knows the answer they assure you there's 'No problem!' to make you feel better while nothing much gets done to alter the basic hopelessness of the situation. But it is also the magic key to a philosophical acceptance, to a different scale of time and values, without which you learn nothing. It was to be the most valuable lesson I learned.

I was very twitchy when I first arrived, anxious not to waste time and anxious that the whole trip would turn out to be a failure. Nothing, of course, had actually been arranged and I didn't really know where to start. All my initial contacts for the first few days led me round in circles and up blind alleys. I was starting to feel desperate. 'No problem!' brought on an attack of mild hysteria. By this time my throat had closed down to a pinhole and I was beginning to get shivery. My temperature rocketed up and I became quite ill with a debilitating virus. I was forced to admit temporary defeat so I let myself be wrapped up, put to bed and surrendered to the miraculous tender loving care of an extended African family household where I was never left alone – someone continuously watched over me, sat by me, washed my sweaty clothes and brought me tea to drink.

I slept on and off for the first thirty-six hours, alternately sweating and shivering. Once I awoke with a terrible fright and leapt bolt upright – a giant cockroach was walking up the side of my face! I flung it to the floor and squashed it with a flip-flop, but for the rest of the night I kept imagining I could hear more scuttling. I was wheezing right down in my lungs and feared the complication of pneumonia – my temperature stayed high, my throat hurt and my nose was blocked up. The antibiotic I was taking didn't seem to be having any effect. There was nothing I could do except stay in bed. It was maddening that none of my mind-over-matter techniques seemed to work at all. It occurred to me that the illness was serving a necessary purpose. Perhaps I could try to welcome and ride with it, acknowledging and accepting the need for it.

On the fourth day the gentle sound of women's voices murmuring and laughing and an appetizing smell from the little charcoal braziers woke me at dusk and I knew the fever had passed. I felt a bit washed out but curiously peaceful. As I lay there I had my first real understanding of a truth I'd known theoretically for some time – the importance and the pleasure of living in the present moment. So much of my life has been spent in anticipation mixed with anxiety about tomorrow, or in nostalgia mixed with remorse about yesterday. Just knowing that the present is all there is means that you have to make the most of it. How lucky to have been afforded the opportunity of experiencing at first hand the enveloping warmth, concern, and kindliness of an African family. Hospitality that puts one to shame when one reflects how little we British allow ourselves to be inconvenienced by the needs of others.

At first I had no idea how many people lived in their little house. All I knew was that they had turfed themselves out of the only decent bed in order to give it to me.

Okay, I said to myself, so whatever happens, happens. Even if I don't find a medicine man I have experienced a powerful example of the healing power of love and care and I've learned something. You usually learn more about life when something goes wrong, and sickness is a good way to learn about healing. I settled down to enjoy my convalescence and the chance to acquire a bit of an insider's view of family life here.

The Twaha family represents a perfect microcosm of contemporary Africa, illustrating all the paradoxes and dilemmas facing a people with one foot in a timeless rural past and the other foot in a high-speed technological future. Ali is a news cameraman for the Voice of Kenya television station. He travels a lot and has a wide experience of the outside world. He also seems to know everyone and acts as a liaison person, interpreter and fixer for visiting film crews. He is father and provider for his whole vast elastic family network – very generous and good-natured.

Maryam is his wife and the central pivot of the household. She works all day as a catering assistant at the police headquarters and spends the rest of the time cooking and caring for her family. She reminds me of a mother cat with a large litter of kittens – soft and gentle really but very sharp-tongued – everyone jumps to her commands. The older boys wouldn't dream of smoking or drinking in front of her and the little ones don't squabble when she's around. She is devoted to her kids and hates to be away from home where she can't keep an eye on them. Unfortunately, as she doesn't speak any English and I don't speak Swahili we could only converse through other members of the family.

They have six children of their own, ranging in age from twenty-five down to ten, who all live at home (unemployment among young people is a serious problem here too) and all have learned English at school. Another son died tragically some years ago from a food-poisoning accident at his school. They also have two adopted children, one beautiful six-year-old girl whose mother is mentally ill and cannot look after her and another darling child, my own special favourite, Fauzia, ten years old and suffering from a cruel crippling disease. The Twahas took her in out of pity when she was rejected by her own family. She is a brave and much-loved member of the clan.

Maryam's youngest sister, Tijara, a secretary, also lives in the house, as do three teenage nieces who earn their keep by helping with the chores. Apart from the permanent residents, any number of neighbours' kids, friends and relatives constantly throng in and out. The house consists of a comfortable sprawl of six small rooms around a central courtyard. This is the hub of all activity – everything goes on in the courtyard: cooking, washing, sitting around, visiting, talking, feeding babies, break-dance practising, hair-plaiting. They all bunked up together while I had the only double bed to myself. They got quite upset when I protested so in the end I shut up. I can't believe there can possibly be a word for 'privacy' in the Swahili language. The concept just doesn't seem to exist. They thought it was very odd of me to want to go off and write in my journal on my own. Usually a couple of people would come and keep me company.

95

Because of Ali's relatively secure job, the family are better off than most of their neighbours. They have a proper toilet and shower, a television, a video, and a battered old Renault, but that's where the luxury ends. As an ordinary working-class family they have far fewer material things than their British counterparts. Their only indulgence is to hire two video films a week and watch them on a Saturday night. Everyone has to be fed every day, school fees found, shoes, books, and school uniforms bought, bills paid, poorer relations helped, family obligations honoured. It's a hard life and yet they made room for me so cheerfully and open-heartedly.

Food is always sufficient, if carefully eked out, but there are never any treats – only essentials. They make a very little meat go a long way, chopped small and added to a vegetable stew for flavour. Everyone keeps urging me to eat more but, conscious of how many people there are to feed here, I'm eating much less than I usually do. It's a very healthy diet, tasty and nutritious. No sugar, no junk or additives, no animal fats except a bit of ghee, plenty of fresh fruit, vegetables and, of course, fibre in the form of the staple filler ugali, or rice, or chapattis.

The chapattis are especially delicious but very time-consuming to prepare. It would drive me crazy, I'm so programmed to get on, finish my work and *then* relax. Nobody here seems to mind that the cooking and washing take all day. In fact they are regarded more as social occasions to be enjoyed than dreary tasks. Pleasure is taken in the job itself rather than in its completion. During the week the three teenage girls, Ayuma, Mamu and Zuhura scrub, sweep, and prepare the evening meal, but on Saturday all the women do it together – including me while I was there – it is a time for gossip and chat, laughter and stories.

The day begins at 6 am when three little charcoal braziers are lit to heat the washing water. There is a mountain of washing to be done so everyone takes a little low wooden stool and a bucket of suds and we sit around in the courtyard in the fresh morning sunshine scrubbing away.

They were all very curious about English family life and bombarded me with questions, laughing with embarrassment as they blurted out the more personal ones: 'Do English husbands beat their wives?' they wanted to know. I told them that domestic violence is much more widespread than most people want to admit but that we do have refuges where battered wives can find protection. Everyone thought that was a marvellous idea but doubted whether it would catch on in Kenya. African women, I was told, have a pretty raw deal on the whole, are still treated as property with very few legal or financial rights and in country areas can still be bought and sold for a few goats . This, of course, is changing, but they are still very far behind us in the area of emancipation and equality. Ali is an exceptionally kind and loving father and husband and I never saw even a hint of violence in their home but I gather that's quite rare. What isn't at all rare is the distinctly dual standard of morality between the sexes.

What would Maryam do, I wanted to know, if Ali announced he was taking another wife? As a Muslim he is entitled to four. 'She would die the same day!' snarled Maryam in reply, eyes narrowing to little slits. I believed her.

They couldn't believe stories they'd heard of cruelty to children in Britain and America. 'Do parents really harm their own children?' I was asked. I had to admit that child abuse was unfortunately quite common. They were astonished. I never saw a child cry in Kenya for longer than it took for someone to rush over and pick it up. Parents are endlessly indulgent and physically affectionate and elder children patient and protective with the little ones. They delight in their children and there is also a clear-cut code of respect for elders so it would be unthinkable for kids to be disobedient or cheeky. What a shame we seem to have lost that equilibrium. Our other great failure, of course, is with the integration of old people in our society. My friends were thunderstruck at the thought of retirement homes or geriatric hospital wards. In an extended family system everyone always has a home, companionship and a useful role to play. Maryam's mother lives up the road. A round, hobbly, grumbly old lady wrapped up in two kangas. She just waddles in with a couple of cronies and sits on the wall. Some of the babies climb on her. Nobody says much, no great greetings, they just acknowledge her presence and giver her a corncob to eat. When her time comes she will die naturally with the people she knows around her and not have her life endlessly prolonged by modern drugs.

'What would I do if an older son came home with VD?'
'What would I do if my daughter got pregnant?'
'What would I do if my husband took a mistress?'
'What kind of food would I cook for a special feast?'

We talked and talked, shared worries and wisdom and old wives' tales and learned much about each other's lives.

They have, in fact, got an ancient twin-tub washing machine but they don't like using it because it's 'too lonely'.

The sun shone, the jacaranda filled the air and I felt much better.

Saturday is also the day Maryam and Tijara go shopping at the market. I asked if I could go along. They laughed but took me anyway. Ali drove us in his old banger to the main produce market on the outskirts of Nairobi. I could see why they were surprised I wanted to come. The place is a nightmare crush of bodies and lorries and mountains of fruit. It's so slippery underfoot from a carpet of squashed rotting pineapples and other assorted fruits that one is constantly in danger of falling and never being able to get up again. I was terrified I would lose sight of my protectors as the only, suddenly very conspicuous, outsider in a sea of shouting, shoving buyers and sellers. Porters bent double under enormous sacks of potatoes barged past whistling for people to get out of the way. People staggered under impossible loads like beasts of burden. Luckily, Maryam was sporting a day-glo pink chiffon headscarf so I could see her bobbing along in front. The heat was terrible and all the noise, confusion, filth and diesel fumes unbearable. Maryam only bought two kilos of peas and a bunch of coriander leaves. All that awful hassle to save a few pence was a salutary reminder of how carefully she has to budget. We stopped at other little stalls selling this and that – a bunch of bananas, a sack of potatoes, some mangoes, etc., and gradually the week's supplies were collected.

From about 3 pm onwards the great cooking marathon starts.

Everyone cooks, not just one poor harassed mother slaving over the kitchen stove. It's very companionable and unhurried, a few charcoal braziers in the courtyard and each woman sitting on a little stool stirring or chopping, peeling or frying. At one point the boys gave us an impromptu demonstration of their latest body-popping and break-dance routine. Break-dancing has taken the younger generation by storm and the smash-hit film in Nairobi, retained by popular demand, is *Beat Street*. The tinny tranny belted out Herbie Hancock's 'Rocket Man' and the lads jerked into action. The older boys were sensational, flipping and roboting and spinning round on their heads while the little guys with their skinny, flailing legs looked more like stick insects or electrocuted spiders trying to copy their big brothers. It was very touching to watch, but also sad to see the way in which this aggressive, pulsating, imported American culture creates a restless dissatisfaction with their own traditions and whispers promises of excitement and unfulfilled longings that can only bring in their wake the destruction of all that this timeless firelight circle stands for.

The cooking took four hours, the meal was eaten in five minutes. After dinner the men usually watch the football on television and then go out – nobody asks where. The women crowd into the video room, wrap themselves up in their kangas and watch the videos. This Saturday the programme consisted of two unspeakable video nasties that would almost certainly be banned in this country. Fortunately the quality of these fourth-hand pirate copies is so bad that it's nearly impossible to tell what's going on. The women all chew leaves with a mild stimulant effect so that they can make the most of Saturday night, stay awake till dawn and sleep tomorrow. Everyone nattered away cheerfully while heads rolled on the screen. I felt quite upset and ashamed about this example of Western 'culture'. What a legacy to give anyone! What can they make of it all? I could only stomach five minutes of the first one and took the little children off to show them how to make a game of Snakes and Ladders.

Tijara decided I should have my hands decorated in the style of a Swahili bride. She mixed up a paste of henna powder, hot water and lemon juice then, using a matchstick, carefully painted an elaborate design on my palms and fingernails. Then I had to hold my hands above the heat from the charcoal brazier until the paste had dried. The whole process took about two hours and I had to sleep with the dried paste intact which was extremely difficult. Undoing my bra strap, turning back the sheets and trying to read a few pages of my book were major manœuvres, with bits of crumbling clay getting everywhere. I slept like a dead possum with my hands in the air.

I suppose the person I came closest to during my convalescence was Tijara and I felt the poignancy of her predicament acutely. As a single career girl who loves Mills and Boon romantic novels, *True Love* magazine stories and funky disco music she has very Western expectations and longs to make the transition to 'modern woman', although at home she conforms to the traditional fireside pattern and wants to get married and have children. She is very pretty, with a radiant face, beaded hair and classic Kikuyu looks. More than anyone else in the family she has a foot in both camps – kanga at home, glitter sweater and hot pants at the disco. Her most precious possession is her *Jane Fonda Workout Book* and I've promised to send her the proper gear with leg-warmers, etc. so she can look the part.

When I finally felt strong enough to get back on the trail again Ali took me to the offices of *The Nation*, one of Kenya's daily newspapers, to see if they had any library material on traditional doctors. I spoke to a young reporter who remembered an article on the work of Dr John Muia Kalii, an Akamba man from the Machakos district in the Eastern Region. He had many miraculous cures ascribed to him and was held in some awe by the local people. The article described the successes he had had with mental illness and infertility.

Only an hour later I was talking to a woman writer who had just published a book on heroic Kenyan women. When I asked her if she knew any healers she immediately spoke of 'a remarkable man near Machakos called Kalii'! He had cured her sister, who for years had suffered from suicidal depressions. She had been lethargic, negative and anxious, now she was well and leading a normal life.

That same evening at dinner, a Ugandan refugee paediatrician working at the Kenyatta Hospital told me, 'If you are researching healing you must try to locate a certain Dr Kalii. He has an extraordinary knowledge of plants and herbs and has become quite a legend in his own lifetime.'

Three references in one day. I couldn't ignore it. Kalii was obviously the chap I was meant to see. He has a little 'hospital' about seven miles off the main Nairobi–Mombasa highway where he treats patients for a wide variety of physical and mental disorders, many of which have been declared incurable by conventional doctors. I also heard that apart from speaking no English he has a reputation for being a bit prickly with snooping outsiders whom he suspects of trying to steal his secret potions and claim the credit for his life's work.

There was no way to inform Kalii of my intended visit but Ali and Maryam came up with rather a good plan: since they both had long-standing unresolved medical problems they would go there as patients, bringing me along as a friend. I could introduce myself, find an interpreter, and stay on as long as I wanted, making my own way back afterwards. Maryam was a bit nervous for my welfare but I reassured her that so long as I took a mosquito net and continued to feel all right I should be okay. It certainly seemed as good a plan as any. I felt as if the week of forcibly having to wind myself down to a more philosophical acceptance of life as it comes had prepared me in the best possible way for what was to follow. I also felt strangely protected in some way, open, trusting, and above all curious.

We left Nairobi for the two-hour drive through green undulating plains dotted with trees and the occasional giraffe or ostrich posing as if they'd been paid by the Kenya Tourist Board. In Machakos, a small provincial town, we looked up a friend of Ali's, the young *Nation* correspondent based here, and he brought along Calvin, who apparently knows Dr Kalii well and even, as it transpired later, is planning to marry one of his daughters who is expecting Calvin's baby! Calvin is a fat jolly guy who got a bit tiresome as the evening wore on and he downed several pints of beer at my expense. He spent a lot of time telling me how well he knows the old man and how much he, Calvin, is accepted as one of the family. He was a bit shifty so I hoped it wasn't all bullshit. We agreed a £50 interpreter's fee which was just about all the money I had.

I tried to convey to Calvin that my intentions were serious and genuine. I stressed that I did not want to pick the doctor's brains nor steal his secrets but humbly to observe, possibly help, and learn what it is about him that makes him a good healer. I don't think Calvin really got the message. As the evening grew darker he began to tell me hair-raising stories about other shamans living in the area. There is a witchdoctor who lives nearby, a very powerful man able to bewitch even other witches. He gains possession of their magic spells and throws them into the Indian Ocean, he urinates on the heads of those who don't cooperate. It is rumoured that human skulls and genitals have been found near his hut . . .

There is also, he told me, a local man who specializes in snake-bite cures made from snake gall or crushed snakeskulls or something, and yet another who can put a death curse on someone from which it is impossible to recover. The point of these blood-curdling tales, I think, was to make me feel grateful to have Calvin's protection. Certainly I had no idea what to expect from Kalii and confess to having felt a little bit apprehensive at that stage, especially since so few people speak English. Calvin's isn't all that great and I wasn't sure I'd really managed to get across the sincerity and simplicity (naivety) of my purpose. Unfortunately, to many Africans, a European woman is either a bossy memsahib to whom you act dumb and reveal nothing, a rich tourist to rip off, or someone to take revenge on for past colonial humiliations by exercising your new power and arrogance. I just wanted Kalii to like and trust me.

In the meantime I rented a room in the T-Ten Hotel in Machakos for forty shillings: a little concrete cell with a barred window, a bed with sheets, a toilet and a cold tap, a table and chair, and a Gideon Bible. The walls were stencilled all over in an attempt at home-made wallpaper and in the middle of one wall was the legend: 'CAUTION! Whatever is in this room is

CLEAN. Please keep it same. Thanks by Management.' In fact it was pretty clean – no flies, no smell. Downstairs there was a little restaurant selling chicken stew and chapattis, very tasty and good value for eighteen shillings with a cup of boiled tea.

The next day we would confront the formidable Mzee Daktari, the 'old man doctor' as he is respectfully known.

We made our pilgrimage to the 'hospital' first thing in the morning. It is a collection of mud-walled shacks with corrugated roofing set under wide-spreading flame trees in a large compound of red earth, dry and dusty from the drought. Mzee Daktari was sitting under a tree talking to a patient when we arrived and came forward to greet us courteously, sending a child to fetch glasses of water to revive us after the journey. He is a tall imposing figure with the limpid eyes, drooping upper lip and gentle quizzical expression of a giraffe. Nothing could have been further from the Hollywood image of a juju man with a bone through his nose and feathers in his hair. Here was a very dignified, if rather overweight, figure, neatly dressed in a white coat, collar and tie.

He invited us into his consulting room and arranged himself behind a table piled high with several enormous leather-bound ledgers containing the names of all his past patients. Behind him in the dingy little room was a glass-fronted cabinet with hundreds of little newspaper-wrapped parcels of herbal remedies carefully stacked under their appropriate labels: 'Uterine Failure', 'Falling Hair', 'Syphilis', 'Sex Power' . . . He listened attentively while I was introduced and my friends related their symptoms to him. Ali has some form of dormant leukaemia. Dr Kalii said confidently that his greatest success rate is with cancers of all types. He gave Ali a preparation of powdered leaves to sniff up his nostrils until he sneezed mightily. Now he had to make an infusion of different herbs and drink the liquid three times a day for three weeks and he would be completely cured. No alcohol allowed.

Next Maryam had an examination. She suffers from a chronic gynaecological condition that causes her quite a lot of pain. Kalii held her abdomen carefully for some time with his eyes closed. 'Blocked Fallopian tubes,' he pronounced, and gave her lots of little packets of dried dusty rootsy stuff to be added to boiling water and taken internally. Kalii stood up and hung an old stethoscope around his neck (a gift, I found out later, from a grateful patient), signifying that the consultation was over and my friends left for the journey home.

Now I was on my own. I'd had my doubts about Calvin all along, an uneasy suspicion that he never really had my best interests at heart. When we'd first arrived the Doc had seemed quite amiable about my staying but now Calvin took him aside for a hasty consultation and to my dismay Kalii suddenly demanded a lot of money for his cooperation. He said I would be taking up his valuable time, he had patients waiting to be seen and he couldn't be expected to waste time telling some perfect stranger his secrets. Calvin, the rat, had obviously misrepresented me. I just managed to flag down Ali before he drove off, to intervene on my behalf. 'Please tell him', I implored, 'that no one is funding me, I don't have any money, I come only in a spirit of fellowship and genuine enquiry, I don't want to take up one minute of his time, only to sit in the corner of his consulting room to see what happens and ask him the occasional question about treatment and diagnosis.' Then I played my trump card. 'If he wouldn't be offended could I offer him a gift I have brought?' I produced a rather flamboyant old uncut raw amethyst cluster ring of mine from Mexico which I'd thought might come in handy. It fitted Kalii's little finger exactly and he was clearly delighted. I explained that many people believed amethyst crystals augmented healing power, and that wearing the ring might help him. I showed him my mother's one that I always wear. His mood changed dramatically and from then on I think I was unequivocally accepted. Calvin shrugged his shoulders and grinned as if to say 'It was worth a try'. So long as I remembered not to trust him further than I could throw him, I think we understood each other reasonably well from then on.

Doc took me on a tour of his 'wards': three scruffy little shacks with corrugated-iron roofs. Two were empty except for a litter of kittens and a few goats, but the third room had four mattresses on the floor and four women patients. They had been there for varying lengths of time. One had come in with jaundice, a very distended swollen liver and yellow eyes, he said. She had been there two weeks; he had me feel her abdomen to see how the swelling and tenderness had gone. Another was a sweet little woman in her early forties with greying hair. She told me she had been married since 1956 and failed to become pregnant in all that time. She had tried everything and finally come to Kalii as a last resort when she heard of his reputation with infertility. He had treated her and she had returned to her village. Now she was here to show him she was five months pregnant. She pressed my hands to her tummy and I felt the baby move. Her face was radiant and she was knitting a little garment in fluorescent green wool.

There was an elderly lady who'd had cataracts in both eyes and been growing progressively blind for years. Her sight was now restored and her eyes looked pretty clear to me considering her age. The last young woman had a heart problem. Her heart had been beating very fast; she had high blood pressure with swollen puffy limbs and too much water retention. She looked as right as rain after twenty-four hours and a dose of herbal medicine. As he talked about each one he sat by her on the bed with a hand on her head or holding her arm. The strongest message he was projecting was one of care and compassion. A non-judgemental, parental sort of love. The patients obviously adore him and he transmits a quiet air of life-affirming hope.

I was still bothered by a miserable hacking cough left over from the flu. Doc looked at me in amusement as I spluttered and wheezed. He just motioned for me to follow him and we went back to his consulting room. He called his youngest wife to bring a glass of water (always boiled and filtered, he asserted), sprinkled a pinch of something from one of his little packets, swilled it round until the water turned reddish brown then bade me drink the bitter liquid. It burned a bit going down but my throat almost instantly felt better, less raspy and tickly. From the taste, which reminded me of a Fisherman's Friend lozenge, I would guess it contained liquorice root, pepper, menthol and gum arabic. I asked him what was in it and he smiled enigmatically so I gave him one of the lozenges from my handbag to taste and he laughed heartily as he recognized the similarity. He couldn't quite believe my nerve. I didn't cough again even once after taking his remedy.

Patients arrive at any time throughout the twenty-four hours. Some have walked for days to get here and the little verandah is constantly crowded with patients and their families waiting to see Mzee. There has been an attempt to make the place look smart by painting whitewash on the stones lining the driveway but the general air is of a run-down dilapidated sprawl. A grateful rich ex-patient has built him a dam and a generator so there is never a shortage of water or electricity. The area of land he owns has been added to in order to be self-sufficient in crops, to feed the resident patients and the large extended family he supports. He has three white-coated trainee helpers on the premises but today they were sleeping because they had been on night duty.

It is rumoured that some Very Important People indeed come and consult the Daktari under cover of darkness, not wanting to be thought backward or superstitious. It's still not considered very modern or sophisticated for government ministers and the like publicly to endorse this kind of thing. Even the late Jomo Kenyatta's name is reputedly in the leather-bound ledger, although Kalii quite rightly refused to confirm this in the name of professional confidentiality.

From what I gathered in Nairobi, people are gradually becoming more confident about acknowledging the value in some of the indigenous health practices. The world is getting smaller all the time. Colonial arrogance about 'primitive beliefs' and local methods is much less prevalent than it used to be. Many Western-trained doctors and psychiatrists have come to understand the immense importance of learning to utilize and integrate folk-healing and shamanic practices before they are lost forever. The witchdoctor (a title often misused), native doctor, herbalist, tribal medicine man — repositories of ancient wisdom — have come to be seen as an essential adjunct to a comprehensive and workable health care scheme in developing countries. The World Health Organization actively encourages the cooperation of orthodox medical practitioners and local healers. It would like to see a gradual synthesis of traditional values and wisdom with the advances of modern science and technological know-how.

Kalii's therapeutic style is very paternalistic and incorporates his personal idiosyncrasies. He is not troubled by uncertainties or doubts and has a well-defined professional style. One of the essential ingredients of his success is the fact that his little hospital is small and homely and located near to the people it serves. It is open house at all times and patients do not feel alienated by the surroundings. It looks like home – animals, children, cooking going on. Patients have their personal belongings with them and relatives are encouraged to stay and help with caring for them.

That first evening, a madman came into the compound – raving and filthy, waving a stick and shouting at everybody. Barking, snarling dogs surrounded him. The children laughed and ran away. He had obviously been on the road a long time, rejected and cast out by society, moved on by every village. Kalii went out, sat down and shared his food with him. He held his hand, they talked and laughed. The incident had a biblical simplicity and fundamental symbolism about it. Finally Kalii drove the man home to his village in his own car. It must have been a long way off because he didn't come back until long after I left.

I had decided to rent a little room in Salama, the original one-horse truck-stop town back down on the highway. I could have stayed at Kalii's place but I didn't want to be a drain on their limited resources – also I knew that a bit of privacy occasionally would be a blessed treat. Doc has promised me a driver to fetch me in the morning.

Salama is a dump! A string of one-storey shop fronts, mostly bars, dance halls, eating places and knocking shops with barefoot hookers in faded frocks hoping to earn the price of a bowl of stew. Frequented by long-distance lorry drivers, the place is alive with activity at night. Marvellously evocative East African music coming from the juke box and a great deal of squeaking bedsprings in the next cubicle to mine carried on till the sound of fifty long-haul truck engines warming up in the dawn light heralded the departure of the men on their way from Mombasa to Uganda. Everyone washed and peed right outside my little cell window at about 5 am before the mass exodus of monstrous motors.

In the morning the promised vehicle failed to arrive so I sat fretting for a while until I realized what a useless activity that is and what an inappropriate response to the vicissitudes of African life. The 'Christ! Let's get things moving' attitude of northern Europeans is looked upon with great puzzlement by people who spend a lot of time sitting around enjoying the communal pleasures of just chewing the fat. In Salama, though, the ennui and inertia that pervades everything seems more highly magnified. I guess that's the nature of a truck-stop town. People sit and wait for customers, wait for a bus, wait for a truck to be fixed, wait for news, wait to shine shoes or sell mangoes. People dressed in indescribable rags prop up doorways and wait for handouts. The local sharp lads in threadbare flares and down-at-heel seventies platform shoes wait for the action. Calvin, chewing a matchstick, had been hoping to pick up some cut-price local talent but the girls were all exhausted. He is a companion of limited interest so to avoid having to make conversation I bought the *Kenya Times* to read over a breakfast of fried buns and boiled tea. I read the following riveting piece of information: 'Cockroaches are an important ingredient in folk-medicine. Mashed in sugar they can be applied to cancer sores or ulcers to help them heal. A mixture containing cockroach ashes can be drunk to kill worms. In powder form cockroaches can be used as medicine for dropsy. Fried in oil with garlic, cockroaches can be eaten to aid digestion.' And to think I squashed one!

Queues of women with babies on their backs wait in the sun for the matatus (communal taxis) to take them about their business, a mangy dog waits in the middle of the road, fruit sellers with piles of pomegranates sit under trees knitting cheap fluorescent lime-green wool into tea-cosy hats for their babies. Finally our transport arrived at noon. The driver had run out of petrol *and* got a puncture. Back at the hospital, Doc, who had been up all night sitting with the family of the deranged man, had only just woken up anyway. He invited me into his consulting room again and we talked a lot about the counselling aspect of his work. Many patients come to him complaining of being bewitched or possessed. As a Christian himself he encourages them not to believe in witchcraft. Nobody can be bewitched who doesn't believe in it, he says; the power of God is far stronger and love can always conquer fear. This is what he told the poor madman's family. He sees himself as being a conduit to God, and a channel for the divine force that does the actual healing work.

Men often come to him suffering from impotence. He says it is very rarely a physical problem but rather a mental one, where the man has feelings of inferiority and anxiety about not measuring up or of losing his wife to another man. Doc insists on seeing the couple together, and tells the man to show more love to his wife. He advises them to try and be alone, to play together and 'enjoy each other very much'. He gives them both potions to take: one for the man, to make him 'strong all the night and never go down', one for the woman to make her 'equal to his power'. An enlightened approach in a part of the world where men are men and don't usually feel they have to waste time with the subtleties of technique. Kalii was watching how I took all this talk about sex. When he was satisfied that I could keep my cool he cracked a few ribald jokes and laughed his head off. He discourages female circumcision, he told me, because it diminishes sexual response in women, which would be a bad thing. For a couple to remain happy and a husband really to enjoy sex with his wife, she should derive pleasure and satisfaction from the experience as well. I agreed heartily.

He highly recommends his 'Sex Power for Men' medicine, especially for 'old' men of his age who have married younger women. He is fifty. His new young wife came into the room looking sleek and sly. She is the one entrusted with the secret recipe so that she can manufacture the supplies of this potion for him. She gave him a knowing glance and he ran his hand affectionately down her ripening front. She is pregnant and they plan to have five children, he says. He had seven with his first wife, who died, and has five with his second. He supports the whole lot cheerfully and is teaching the wisdom and secrets of his calling to two of his children. One daughter in particular has an aptitude for the work. She is sixteen and very smart and he holds out high hopes for her. He's promised to give me some of his virility potion to take home to my husband if I can stand the pace! He's obviously a sexy old thing and this talk cleared the air a bit and got our relationship on to a more bantering and informal plane. He still couldn't quite understand what I was doing travelling around Kenya on my own without the protection of a man.

As we were talking the door flew open and a young woman staggered in doubled over with pain. She fell gasping on the examination bed, her anxious relatives hovering nearby. Kalii gently patted and massaged her, talking to her in a reassuring quiet voice. He stroked her arms and gave her a dose of some dried roots and bark. 'Appendix,' he told me without hesitation. If it was an acute case and the appendix was about to burst, he says, he would still treat her but then get her to hospital as quickly as possible. The same with anything infectious like TB. He believes in close cooperation with the medical profession, but prefers to try to avoid cutting or harming the body in any way. In this instance he decided he had caught it early enough. He told me the medicine would fizz out all the bits of muck – particles of rice, stones, fingernails, dirt – from the dead-end trap in the gut. The area should then be left clean with no need for surgery. Her relatives helped her back to a chair in the waiting room and within an hour I saw her setting off jauntily for the six-hour walk back to her village, laughing and waving.

Another woman arrived with a hideous disfiguring tumour on the side of her face, a painful growth inside her mouth on her palate, and a lump on her breast. She had been in hospital in Nairobi and they had told her it was too far gone to operate and there was nothing further they could do. She was twenty-eight years old and they had sent her home to die. Kalii practically rubbed his hands with glee. Terminal cancer was his speciality, he said, and he'd never lost a patient yet.

He gave her one of his herbal concoctions, laid her down on the table and held his hands on and around her face. She was quite dirty and sweaty and he tenderly wiped her temples with the corner of her kanga. She looked very ill, with an awful grey complexion, more dead than alive. I wouldn't have thought she had much of a chance. As he worked he explained that the power in his hands is what disperses tumours and relieves pain. The power comes directly from God and he is only God's tool. The girl visibly relaxed and her expression became more peaceful as he stood with closed eyes, his great bulk three times her size towering over her, and ministered to her with infinite gentleness.

She was taken away by her family and given a cot in one of the wards. When I looked in on her later, she was huddled under some threadbare rags, asleep. It didn't seem possible that she could recover. I asked Kalii how he acquired his power and he told me that ever since he was a child he knew he was different. His mother and his grandmother before him were both village sorceresses. He is the only male in the family to have inherited the gift and although it is a great responsibility he never gets tired because God, he says, also gives him the energy to do His work.

It is interesting to me to reflect that for thousands of years in Europe or here people had but one healer, the sorceress. Everyone consulted the wise woman. If her cure failed they abused her and called her a witch. Held in awe and made a scapegoat, a user of herbs and potions to heal and save – she was both needed and feared. She who worked so many miracles and soothed so much human agony was the martyr of the Middle Ages. But the sorceress has not perished forever in the West and has remained pretty constant in Africa – a sort of hereditary divine priesthood is usually passed on down the female line because nurturing, pity, compassion, gentleness, have traditionally been thought of as feminine qualities, though not exclusively feminine – bearers of light can be of either sex but perhaps healing flourishes better in a society where the female principle is well integrated.

There are 3,885 different herbs in Doc's repertoire. I am sure some of them have efficacious properties but I'm equally sure that it is the man himself with his simple unhurried kindliness who is the healing catalyst. He says he can tell what's wrong with a person by 'reading' their blood. He takes hold of an arm and feels with both hands up and down, sometimes pressing his ear to the inside of the wrist or elbow. This seems to be a process of attunement similar to that which I've learned from other healers (using the pendulum or scanning the chakras): aligning your own intuition and sensitivity to the patient's needs. Kalii closes his eyes and appears to go into himself for the answer he seeks. He doesn't really have the words to explain what is happening but says he just 'knows'. In his dreams he often sees the right herbal preparation to give for a particular ailment.

This provided interesting links with the techniques of inner journeys, visualizations, inspirational guidance and extended sensory awareness that I have been learning about wherever good healing goes on. 'Once you have found the way you will never lose it,' he told me. 'But the power is enormous — delicate and dangerous. If I ever tried to use this power against an enemy, I would be caught in the trap of evil.' He also warned me not to speak indiscriminately of these things but to learn to keep my counsel. 'Then you will become more powerful. You will be able to light up and "see" with inner eyes, you will be truly "awake", and your own pains will fall away from you like dead leaves on a tree.' (Old Calvin did rather well here. He usually mangled any poetic explanation to death in the translation.)

Albert Schweitzer once said, 'The witch-doctor succeeds for the same reason all the rest of us succeed . . . we are at our best when we give the doctor who resides within each patient a chance to go to work.' This adds to the evidence that in an altered state of consciousness the mind may be able to will the body's immune system ('the doctor who resides within') back into action. Jump leads again. Kalii is closely linked with the traditional and emotional frames of reference of his patients. A sort of partnership is formed, an alliance with the hidden powers of nature, as the patient entrusts himself to the doctor and the Daktari himself journeys into the clarity of darkness, seeing with his inner eyes.

I sat on the verandah for a while and talked with some of the patients. Many people had just come to greet the doctor or proudly display a new baby after years of infertility (apparently there are dozens of such babies all named after him!). A well-dressed man with an unsightly skin disease was there; he had heard of Kalii from a shoeshine boy in Nairobi. There were cases of rheumatism, polio, eye problems, 'weakness' and 'sickness'. All had heard stories of how similar critical conditions had been cured instantaneously, most had travelled many miles to get here. While we were talking, an anxious-looking Masai man arrived – big extended holes in his earlobes, spear and woolly hat. His wife is one of the barren women Daktari has helped to become pregnant. She wasn't with him because they were afraid it would be dangerous for her to travel. She is in her sixth month and suddenly experiencing pain and bleeding. The husband was distraught and had come to persuade the Doc to visit their village. Kalii agreed at once. Probably only something minor, he guessed, but it was important to reassure the family. He would also take the opportunity to gather some of his wild plants that only come from that area. I was dying to go too but he wouldn't take me; he said it was too far and he would be returning too late.

Everyone piled into the car – he would drop Calvin and me off at our doss house on the way. He insisted on seeing me right to my flea-pit which everyone agreed was a really good room. While the poor Masai waited outside in the car, Kalii bought me a brandy and coke and had a second beer himself. He never drinks in public, so as not to alarm or disillusion his patients. He seemed reluctant for the evening to end and stayed talking for ages. It was frustrating trying to filter my more mystical and philosophical points through Calvin's rapidly deteriorating English (he was now onto his sixth pint). I wanted to communicate some of my thoughts about healing as a transmission of energy and the healer as a vessel through which that energy passes, rekindling the patient's failing recuperative powers.

'Yes! Yes!' Kalii nodded vigorously. Then he grabbed my arms one at a time and felt up and down the main blood vessels. He placed one hand on the top of my chest and felt my hands and wrists. He said I definitely had the temperament and the right blood temperature to be a healer. My hands were full of power, he said, and he would teach me how to read blood tomorrow when I could spend all day at his side. He gave me a great bear hug and disappeared.

Calvin and I ate in a place up the road, the zebra-striped Usalama restaurant, where we ran into Johnny Mulai, a sign-writer and artist who has decorated all the shop fronts here and up and down the length and breadth of Kenya with wonderful lurid designs depicting scenes from rural and urban life, traditional stories or historical events. He is an unusual chap who travels the country plying his trade like an itinerant medieval craftsman.

No car again in the morning! It was supposed to arrive at 8 am but nobody keeps to any prearranged plan. I also got the feeling that I was being tested. One of the subtler aspects of power is how the 'Great One' becomes the centre of his universe – everything revolves around his rather capricious whims, and now I was being made to wait until he was ready. Never mind! Events have their own rhythm here and it's just as well to surf with the tide. I talked to Johnny Mulai instead. He took me round the town to see all the places where he's painted murals – butcher shops with gory carcasses, dance halls with couples in modern fashions doing The Bump. He is a simple, sincere misfit, dressed in ancient clothes and down-at-heel shoes, who carries his paints and brushes wherever he goes roped up in a squashed cardboard box. I especially liked his mural entitled 'You can never escape death!' – a forester being chased by a lion clinging to a rotting branch which is about to break and drop him in the river where a crocodile is waiting. Suddenly I had the idea that since I can't afford to donate any meaningful sum of money to the Doc's establishment, I could offer to commission Johnny (for 300 shillings – about £15) to paint a mural on the hospital wall, showing, perhaps, a downcast sufferer arriving, the Daktari administering his treatment, and the person leaving, happy and cured.

Everyone seemed to think that was an inspired plan, so Johnny waited with us for the transport to arrive. It finally turned up at 1 o'clock. They had a puncture again so we waited another hour for it to be fixed. It's no use being in a hurry here. No sign of

Doc when we arrived; instead we were ushered into his parlour – a grimy room with cement floor, several sagging, dilapidated red leatherette sofas covered with the ubiquitous lime-green crocheted shawls that all the women sit around making, and a photo of Daniel T. Arap-Moi, the President of Kenya. Some old dried faded bougainvillaea flowers had been taped along the picture rail. We sat and sat like a lot of Gumbie cats until suddenly the door opened and lunch appeared. Kalii joined us but hardly spoke to me. After his effusive behaviour the night before he was distinctly cool. I couldn't even find out what had happened to the Masai wife yesterday. I felt very uneasy and not at all sure what his game was. A grateful young woman patient had travelled a very long way to greet him. She had been in Sweden where the best Scandinavian doctors and specialists had failed to cure her of terrible recurring infections and inter-uterine pain. She felt sure that all the tablets and pills were poisoning her body and creating side-effects even worse than her original complaint. So she had come home and placed her trust in a system she felt suited her better. 'Africans should only take boiled herbs from their own country,' she told me. Everyone was amazed to see her happy smiling face and healthy demeanour, remembering her as a thin miserable girl racked by years of suffering.

I introduced Johnny and Kalii seemed pleased enough with the suggestion of the mural, but a little while later there was an unpleasant incident when Calvin translated to me, 'The doctor says, if you can afford to pay the artist, why can't you afford to pay some more money for my expenses?' I was absolutely sure the doctor said no such thing. Calvin was just stirring things up again. I got a bit fed up and put the 300 shillings on the table, saying, 'This is all I have. If you'd rather use it for petrol or anything else instead of a mural, just do what you want.' Kalii immediately called in Johnny and handed him the money. Then ensued a lengthy discussion of how the Doc was to be portrayed. He dug out lots of photos of himself and selected the most flattering so that Johnny could get the likeness right. Alas, I would never see the mural completed.

A car-load of rich merchants from Mombasa arrived. More

grateful ex-patients, I was told, come to pay their respects. They sat and waited, patients sat and waited, we sat and waited. Doc moved slowly, walking around with the air of someone who never does the waiting and accepts without question the devotion of his milieu. He really was being infuriating that day.

I went over to the ward to see how Zakia, the cancer patient, was doing and was astonished to see the lump on the side of her face had shrunk to half the size! I asked Kalii if I could sleep up at the hospital for the remainder of my time. Their transport system is so unreliable and I couldn't bear to fritter away another day with waiting. At least on the premises I would have some control over events. Another day in Salama would have driven me barmy.

I made myself a little nest in the corner of one of the empty 'wards'. But some time in the middle of the night a family came in with a young man having terrible convulsions. I only had my torch to see by but it looked to me as though he was in an epileptic fit. I remembered two bits of folk wisdom from my mother which were: Hold the person's tongue to stop them choking to death, and try to stop them injuring themselves. I did both those things in the absence of any other remedy, and then just placed my hands on him in what I hoped would be calming and soothing places until he became quiet. I couldn't understand a word of what the man's relatives were telling me and they didn't know what I was doing sleeping on the floor so it was all a bit bizarre. The young chap finally slept, exhausted, and an old lady in the group sang a praise song to me and kept kissing my hands. When Kalii returned after midnight from some visit he'd gone on, he hurried straight along to the ward. He 'read' the patient's blood by the light of a hurricane lamp. He listened with his ear pressed against the man's temple and said, 'You can hear the disease making a noise like insects.' I listened but couldn't hear anything. What I *did* feel was a strong electrical current giving off irregular pulses. I told the Doc what I'd done and he said 'Good'. I felt so chuffed with the praise, such as it was, and realized how hurt I'd really been by his rejection. Pathetic!

I asked him what he called the disease and he said 'power

failure'. The treatment was to draw away the bad energy and to give an infusion of boiled herbs. Everyone settled down and we tried to get some sleep but it was only an hour or so before the sun rose. In the morning I went in to see Zakia. The swelling inside her mouth had completely gone, the lump on her breast had vanished and the growth on her face was now only a quarter of the size! It was absolutely astonishing and I never would have believed it possible. She was sitting up in bed sipping a little tea and managed a wan smile.

More praise from Kalii when I saw him later. 'If you are put here on Earth to cure people, you must never say "No",' he said. 'You did not refuse, you are a good woman.' He told me that as a youngster, he too had suffered from 'power failure', which had made him fall on the ground and hear the roaring of terrible storms in his head. It's interesting how often healers have been very ill themselves, and during the process of recovery, realize their gift of power for healing others. Kalii had visions and dreams as a child and used the knowledge that came to him to cure his family and schoolfriends.

I loved his phrase about the 'roaring of terrible storms in his head'. It seems as if something has to happen to set in motion our higher faculties – we are making a transition as definite as that between sleeping and waking states, such as happens in scientific intuition, poetic illumination, religious ecstasy. A transition from ordinary wakefulness to a state of awakened consciousness – from ordinary knowing to profound understanding. Sometimes our poor infant brains get a flash of illumination. We see the incomprehensible and there is no language to describe it. We flounder with 'being filled with a great light', 'seeing a great magnificence', 'feeling a great beating of wings', but the words are never equal to the task as soon as they have to express those profound feelings or anything to do with revelation, eternity, time, energy, the essence of man or the nature of God.

There is a terrific acceleration in the mind when the inconceivable becomes possible. Tantalizingly, we seem to be equipped with a capacity for infinite knowledge and in certain conditions we can suddenly apprehend the whole mechanism of life. At other times the mind seems as primitive as a squid trapped in a lobster pot. Perhaps African healers, witchdoctors, shamans, can switch into this mode of inner knowing, the awakened state, without the enormous effort needed to slow down the whirring machinery of the rational, logical mind. Kalii is certainly no great intellectual thinker, he's a natural. His accumulated traditions of magic, ecstatic religious experience and hereditary skills seem to provide him with a method nearly lost in the West (but in the process of being rediscovered by the likes of Bruce MacManaway) of liberating that capacity for inner knowing – 'the doctor who resides within'.

The first patient who came into the consulting room that day was a middle-aged skinny woman with yellow eyeballs. She looked very ill and was shaking with fever. Doc sat back in his chair and said to me, 'You examine her. Tell me what's wrong with her.' It was a bit unfair as I couldn't even ask her what her symptoms were. She spoke a language that Calvin didn't understand. I was totally out of my depth but I thought I couldn't do her any harm by just seeing what I could pick up by a process of focusing and intuition. I stood up and scanned her body for any temperature changes or clues as to where the trouble might be located. The only thing I could feel was a distinct coldness in the area of the heart chakra, but I had no idea what that meant and felt pathetically inadequate in the presence of an emergency of this magnitude. Doc laughed at me and read the woman's blood. 'Pneumonia,' he pronounced with great certainty. He gave her a paste to put on her chest and a supply of newspaper packets of herbs. Her family took her away to rest in one of the wards.

I asked him what he felt about death, and at what stage he would feel it better not to intervene. He said he would always try to save a person's life, he would hold out hope and prescribe medicine no matter how critical the condition, but healing could also mean letting go of life happily. 'When God decides, you will know.' He stated his belief in the eternal life of the soul by saying, 'A person's soul does not die. It does not even grow old. An old man still feels young inside because his ageing body has nothing to do with his real self.' Calvin laughed at this. I don't think his mystical side is very highly developed.

The next patient was a very young-looking mother with a very undernourished-looking baby. Doc sent for his senior wife and told her to give the mother some food and to show her how to feed the baby properly. Anyone who comes here looking hungry is always fed first as a matter of course. In fact a large percentage of the problems stems from malnutrition, so food is one of the biggest expenses. Next an old man came in worried about falling hair. Kalii, whose own woolly crop is luxuriant for his age, gave him some potion and some evil-smelling unguent to plaster on the bald patch. I'm sure it was cow dung. Calvin nearly fell off his chair with mirth when the old chap toddled off. There are moments of light relief.

Kalii operates a Robin Hood scale of fees. No one is ever turned away, but the cost of running the place and providing for so many is formidable. Luckily, grateful ex-patients keep on turning up with gifts – a truckful of maize, a supply of fence posts. The parents of an Asian girl gave the hospital a Land Rover after Kalii brought their daughter out of a coma when she had already been certified dead and arrangements were being made for her funeral pyre. Everyone, no matter how illustrious or how unspeakably poor, receives the same individual care. Each is spoken to and listened to with the same attentive gentleness. Our verbal communications were never adequate to describe the subtleties but we developed a pretty close empathy and as I watched him with his patients I think he knew I understood the psychic and spiritual gifts he brought to his work. He gave me some more opportunities to 'read' patients' blood but I didn't really get the hang of it. I don't think the blood itself tells you much but it probably works as a focusing device for the healer's highly developed sensitivity, a method of getting in touch with the healing energy through concentration and compassion.

Zakia's tumour has disappeared! When I saw her she was eating a little rice and vegetables. There was absolutely no sign of it and no scar or distortion. It simply appears to have been re-absorbed by her body. I was so excited to have seen my first real miracle. Nobody else seemed the least bit amazed. Doc was out on a visit that morning, so I had a look at the visitors' book he keeps in his consulting room to see what comments other people have made about him. A party of visiting American doctors had been here and had left effusive remarks in unmistakable American handwriting about his 'magnificent work', his 'true compassion', his 'approach to healing and his love of humanity'. 'Traditional medicines are doing a wonderful job in curing patients,' wrote one. 'Critical conditions recover the very next day,' wrote another. 'God increase his wisdom and bless him in his work.'

It was another one of Kalii's unpredictable days. Since it was to be my last I wanted to see as much as possible but he kept me hanging about for hours. My only defence was not to get rattled. I was sure he wanted to see how far he could push me – whether I would revert to type and pull the impatient white woman stereotype on him. Every African I have met both here and elsewhere on the continent has long memories of insufferable colonial high-handedness. It's very hard to be just a person and not a symbol. Finally, after having virtually ignored me all day he announced I could come with him on safari to a Masai village some two hours' drive away. A few weeks before he had treated a couple of very sick children there who had, he said, diphtheria, and although he was sure there was nothing serious requiring further treatment, he just wanted to visit the family and make sure everything was all right. We piled into the Land Rover with his Rastafarian nephew at the wheel and about eight others in the back with me. We bounced along on spine-jolting metal seats, red dust swirling into our throats and eyes, Doc in the front seat looking magisterial with his stethoscope around his neck. Wherever we went people ran up to the car shouting 'Daktari! Daktari!' Kalii caressed the children's heads, touched and held everyone who came near.

We stopped at a little round mud and straw hamlet where a very old man in rags came hobbling out, both arms uplifted in praise and happiness, to see his beloved doctor. He had been terribly injured in a bus crash which had crushed both his legs.

Doc had treated him after he came out of hospital paralysed and he seemed remarkably spry considering his age and the seriousness of his injuries. Everyone, no matter how ragged or anonymous, is treated with dignity. Although the Daktari is a 'Big Man', in this context he is not overbearing or power greedy. He is the good father, benevolent, caring, shepherding, and he is obviously adored.

The next stop was a hillside full of goats and a few herdsmen. Doc got out and a long appraisal and discussion took place. Suddenly one of the goats was pounced on, tied up and shoved, bleating, into the back of the truck with the passengers, where it butted around frantically, fanned little turds about with its tail, and peed copiously on our feet. No explanation. We lurched on along the rutted dirt road across the invisible border that divides the Masai lands from anyone else's. They had suffered dreadfully in the last year's drought and many of their cattle had died. We drove through one area littered with skeletons every few yards – a vivid reminder of the tenuousness of nomadic life. If the rains fail you starve; it's as simple as that. The Masai are a noble people – nomadic pasturalist herdsmen who have always stubbornly refused to change or fit in with anyone. Successive rulers have singularly failed to make them slaves or soldiers or domestic servants. It's tempting to romanticize them – their knowledge of the wild, their understanding of animals, their elegance and bravery – but the fact is, they haven't sold out – they understand the value of land and they haven't become a miserable, degraded tourist spectacle. People acknowledge and respect their otherness and the integrity which defies intrusion. It's good to see them retaining their dignity, bringing their prehistoric wisdom and customs steadfastly into the twentieth-century city centre while people move over for them – a feat not many so-called primitive cultures have carried off. I heard later that the reason you are forbidden to photograph them in the National Parks is that they actually killed a tourist who ignored their request not to – threw a spear right through him!

The men look very glamorous – tall, fine-featured, with elaborate hairstyles enhanced with red clay. They wear the characteristically draped red cloth or blanket, beaded necklaces, head-bands, bracelets and earrings. They carry spears to defend their cattle against attack by lions and seem to look graceful whatever they do – walking along single file or leaping straight into the air in one of their amazing dances. As we drove along it became dark. African nights descend like a blackout and the Milky Way enfolded us. I'd never seen so many stars near enough to touch, hanging in the trees like diamonds. At last we came to a round fenced enclosure with compact little beehive mud houses, a swept earth compound and a few cows. Lots of delighted children streamed out and some splendidly adorned Masai women, all clamouring to touch their adored Daktari, festooned like Christmas trees with collar-like beaded necklaces and dozens of pairs of beaded hoop earrings hanging from their elongated and perforated earlobes. They mostly have shaved heads and wear colourful red or pink kangas. They look perfect in the landscape but I always found it quite a surprise to see one sitting in a bar with a Coke or speeding by in a taxi in Nairobi. Kalii took my hand and led me doubled over through the spiralling entrance passage of one of the houses. In the absence of a chimney, all the smoke from the fire inside finds its way out through the same passage so I was choking to death by the time I reached the single room inside. An old granny and several others were sitting round the fire cooking something that was sending up clouds of acrid black smoke. I couldn't see much by the light of the single candle and the atmosphere was so intensely suffocating that I had to flee outside again. Everyone laughed at me, the women doubled up with merriment. Mzee Daktari stroked everyone and asked how they were. He read the children's blood and pronounced them completely better. They certainly looked fine. The whole trip seemed more like an excuse for a sociable outing. Doc asked one of the women to go and milk a cow for us, explaining to me that etiquette demands that the visitor must ask – it's not up to the host to offer; then they are happy that your needs have been satisfied. Ten minutes later I was handed an old Mateus Rosé wine bottle corked with a pared-down corncob and filled with fresh foaming warm milk. We sat around in the firelight for a while and a plump, dusty baby climbed into my lap. The mother admired my earrings so I swapped them for a beaded wristband.

Mission accomplished, we piled back in the truck and finally returned to Kalii's little hospital at about 10 pm, where we all solemnly sat around some more in the parlour. Doc then made an elaborate speech to the effect that since I was his honoured guest (he'd hardly spoken to me all day) he intended to throw a farewell party for me. 'There is beer, music, and a goat,' he said with a flourish. My heart sank at the thought of the poor goat. So that was why Doc had acquired it. A party! I hadn't realized I was to be responsible for its execution. Everyone gasped with pleasure and awe at this magnanimous gesture of hospitality and generosity. I knew we'd be in for a long wait as the goat was still protesting in the yard. Ten minutes later when I strolled outside for a breath of fresh air I saw the unfortunate creature strung up by its legs from a tree, being skinned.

A rickety record-player arrived and a handful of scratched 45s – 'Daddy Cool' and about six different Kakamba and Kikuyu songs. Terrific dancing music, and within seconds the room filled up with recuperating patients magnetized by the therapeutic properties of the beat. Crates of beer appeared, donated by some wealthy merchants who'd called earlier in the day. The Doc pulled me to my feet and we initiated the dancing. The old boy was surprisingly nimble and graceful for his bulk and danced like a cross between a potentate and a jelly. Shirt-tails awry, he clasped his belly in both hands and shook it provocatively in my direction. Everyone else instantly joined in until the little room, like a struck tuning fork, began to shimmer and reverberate in the hot equatorial night air. The dancing was wonderful. I don't care if it is a cliché: nobody can dance like Africans. Their bodies set up an undulating wave pattern that just oscillates to the rhythm. It got very sexy and suggestive rather quickly, with everybody laughing and cheering on the ribald gestures of the others. Several of the patients were unstoppable once they got going, especially Zakia, who was poetry in motion, and the yellow-eyed woman with pneumonia. Old Calvin came into his own too, with his overweight, paunchy physique gyrating

123

magically. No one was dressed for a party – they wore just the faded, dusty, raggedy clothes, plastic sandals, and tennis shoes minus laces that they all wear, but it was a great party. Gallons of beer were consumed and the floor was awash with foam.

At one point the good Daktari became alarmingly amorous, as I'd rather feared he might, and started making little speeches about his blood being attracted to my blood and how he'd known it from the first moment he saw me. 'How does it feel to be the guest of honour of our beloved Doctor?' asked one young man pointedly, implying that intense horizontal gratitude should be the appropriate response. 'How do you propose to thank the Doctor when he has killed a goat for you?' was another query. Some delicate negotiations were called for, invoking my jealous husband, my chaste nature, the obligation of hosts to protect lady guests far from home, my untold joyous anticipation at the prospect of being able, some day, to return the generous hospitality in England . . . The situation was reasonably success-fully defused but a watchful attitude was necessary thereafter, like not letting myself get cornered by the doctorial bulk on the sofa.

Everyone was delighted that I ventured to dance in the proper African way and we churned away until three in the morning when the dismembered goat was carried in, done to a turn and piled on several trays. I spared him a guilty vote of thanks for his sacrifice then tucked in. It was not a pretty sight – everyone grabbed handfuls of crunchy intestines, giant knucklebones and ribs, like a scene from Dante's *Inferno*. A mountain of ugali (maize porridge) was consumed and the entire goat, down to his poor little hooves, vanished. Thank goodness Doc's Rasta nephew is a non-drinker since he was the one I hoped would drive me home to my flea-pit. He's a serious good-hearted chap if a bit screwy in his ideas and I was relieved that I could depend on him since everyone else was extremely drunk and the merrymaking looked fit to carry on for days. My erstwhile bodyguard, Calvin, was well away and deeply entangled in what looked like an endless vertical copulation with a young lady so he was in no hurry to leave. The elderly primigravida sitting serenely in the corner, knitting, mostly confined herself to dancing from the waist up, but every once in a while the temptation became too great and she leapt to her feet for a little wiggle. 'Good exercise for the baby,' laughed Doc indulgently. He is convinced that music, laughter and having a good time are an essential part of getting well so parties are a fairly regular feature of hospital life.

Time to make my excuses as a rosy glow suffused the sky. The good doctor gave me a warm embrace and I thanked him for my party and my goat and slipped away. It was 4.30 am by the time Rastaman Martin got me to Salama and the place was completely dead. We had to hammer on the corrugated-iron fence to get the nightwatchman out of bed to let me in. My head was spinning and my throat constricted with dust. I kept doing goat-flavoured burps and one arm was sunburned from leaning out of the truck that day, but I crashed out on my little wooden cot and slept like a log. Calvin staggered in a couple of hours later with two girls and I could hear them heaving about noisily in the next cell.

I'd arranged with Martin to be picked up at 9 am to go and bid a final formal farewell to Doc so I dragged myself up, washed in cold water, and, of course, waited for three hours before he turned up.

Calvin looked very much the worse for wear and poor Martin hadn't been to bed at all. On the drive up to Doc's place for the last time we had a spirited, rather acrimonious argument about the role of women in society. They both conceded that I am an exception (freak?), but they would never marry a 'town woman'; they are all bad. You should never educate an African woman, they said, because she won't stay home and look after her family. Men are superior to women – it says so in the Bible – and women should be able to carry heavy loads on their backs – otherwise it proves they are lazy. 'Why don't you just marry a donkey?' I asked. I think the gulf we were arguing across was too wide for us to have much mutual impact but at least we could laugh at each other. They thought my husband must be an awful wimp to let me go gallivanting off by myself.

Mzee was very happy and expansive and ushered us straight

into his consulting room. He sat himself behind his desk with the leather-bound volumes on it and folded his hands. He said that as a parting present he would like to give me five packets each of his Sex Power for Men and Sex Power for Women medicine to pep up my reunion with my husband. You mix a teaspoon at a time in half a glass of boiling water, cool, strain and drink simultaneously (it's terribly important that one of you doesn't get a head start) before going to bed. 'You will fly,' he guaranteed. 'Your bed will sing, and in the morning you will have to collect your mattress from the other side of the room.' He laughed with bawdy delight at the prospect and I said I could hardly wait since I loved my husband so much.

He solemnly told me that I would be a great healer but I must keep my eyes open, be careful not to be foolishly indiscreet before I am sure I can trust someone, and always to have a loving heart. He marvelled that he'd felt this great empathy with me and was prepared to tell me everything (I don't know how he came to that conclusion; he has refused to divulge even the simplest of his secret recipes). He mentioned that he would like me to arrange a tour of England so he can meet with his medical colleagues and stay with me for two weeks, also perhaps if I could pay his fare . . . Calvin began a bit of free interpretation at this point about how much the doctor was grateful to him for his excellent translating and would be glad if he were to receive a generous present for his services – greedy little sneak! Of course Kalii is a crafty old fox as well and I realize he must be appreciated and understood by a special set of criteria. On one level he is autocratic, pompous, vain, capricious, ignorant and mercenary. At times he can be intolerably rude and insufferably arrogant. But in his role as healer, counsellor, father-figure, provider, saviour, to the thousands of sick, poor, struggling people – mainly peasant farmers – who come to him in need, he is a saint and a miracle worker. A real doctor in a true God-given sense with an uncanny shamanic power, a genius for diagnosis and treatment and a loving heart. We hugged goodbye affectionately and I got a lift back down to Salama.

As soon as I'd given him the agreed fee for his services, Calvin, the rat, jumped on a bus going in the opposite direction and abandoned me to my fate by the roadside. 'No problem!' said someone waiting under a tree, seeing my forlorn look. He flagged down a seven-seater Peugeot with twelve people inside. They all breathed in obligingly, made room for two more and we sped back to Nairobi.

Before returning to England I paid a visit to AMREF, the African Medical Research Foundation, of which the best known section is the legendary flying-doctor service. I wanted to meet Nyambura Githuagui, a senior project worker in health education who has done a lot of sensitive work in an area of great potential value, encouraging cooperation between traditional healers and medical practitioners; acknowledging and respecting the expertise of, for example, traditional birth attendants while at the same time enlightening them on modern methods of hygiene, the importance of using a sterile knife to cut the umbilical cord and of not dressing the wound with fresh cow dung, etc.

She knew of Kalii as she comes from that area but says he is a bit out of the ordinary and much more sophisticated than most. The first of the two main types she has seen in action is the traditional healer (often an old woman), with a calabash full of dried beans and a one-string twangy bow, who sings and chants to a monotonous rhythmic accompaniment until she has transported herself into a state of altered consciousness. Her voice changes, even her language, and she is in touch with her spirit guides who tell her what to do to dispossess the patient – very like the work of trance medium healers in England! The other kind involves a whole group, including the patient. They sing and dance and chant until the patient falls into a trance and is in a blameless state where he is not responsible for his actions, supported by a familiar ritual and spurred on by the non-judgemental acceptance of his peer group – very like the Reverend Jimmie Snow's Evangelical church service in Nashville. While making allowances for obvious cultural variations, the methods used by healers to create a healing space don't seem so very different to me.

Later that day I was asking Sir Michael Wood, founder, director and leading light of the flying-doctor service, what qualities he thinks make a good healer. 'Compassion and a genuine love of people,' he said. ('Love your patients,' was Kalii's answer.) 'They must have confidence and trust in you, and you must acknowledge the whole person, not just the symptoms. In this way you rekindle the life force, and spark the will to live.' 'Mike', as he is universally known, is a wonderful man, adored by his children, his grandchildren and the thousands of shattered lives he has mended with his surgical skills.

His speciality is plastic surgery: the repairing of cleft lip and palate, reconstruction of the damaged hands of leprosy patients, etc. He says modestly that it is the easiest and most rewarding of gifts to bring as an outsider. The results are instantly obvious and people are overjoyed to have a disfigured child handed back to them whole. It also puts people in a better frame of mind to listen to your more general advice on matters of sanitation or family planning – a link with what Elisabeth Kübler-Ross teaches so well: look after the physical needs of your patients first before you presume to counsel or advise.

The flying-doctor service is a marvellous and superbly well-run organization. They do medical and surgical safaris, preventative medicine, first aid and full-scale evacuation missions. They'll fly in and rescue the victims of a road accident, or a tourist taken ill at a lodge. They saved the life of a woman half eaten by lions and a child with meningitis. A plane is always ready to fly, a nurse has an emergency kit prepared in a hangar and they can be airborne in four and a half minutes. They've landed at night with fires along the runway, they've landed on the main Nairobi –Mombasa highway, they've landed on remote tiny airstrips where they've had to buzz elephants off the tarmac.

Mike has good stories to tell of the people he has met in the course of his life out here since 1947. Hemingway was his patient after a plane crash in Tanganyika during the *Snows of Kilimanjaro* days; he once demonstrated a new surgical technique to Schweitzer at Lambarene using only razor blades for the purpose; he played himself in the film *Born Free*. He is a great champion of the idea of an integrated medical service, of the need to study and classify the plants used in herbal medicines, of understanding the cultural elements that apply in curing both physical and mental illness, of undoing the harm of colonial arrogance with its blanket dismissal of anything which didn't conform to Western scientific precepts, and the importance of using all the medical resources at your disposal no matter how unorthodox.

Although their methods and personalities are worlds apart, Michael Wood and John Muia Kalii have some qualities in common. Both are inspired lion-hearted men, both are motivated by love, both are connected to their own inner power and are thus able to work their own kind of miracles.

5

The Truth of Imagination

The intuitive processes in myself have undoubtedly become less creaky as I begin to exercise my mental joints more regularly. This chapter of the story begins with a strange prophetic dream and ends with a startling insight which has enabled me to reclaim and understand a buried bit of my past.

About two years ago I awoke one morning with total recall of a very vivid dream. I had been walking alone along a wide golden shore reminiscent of the Californian beaches of my childhood. The ocean seemed a long way off but the tide was coming in. Cross-currents of shallow translucent water ebbed and flowed over the firm sand. Suddenly, there at my feet, written in the sand, was the name ROSALYN B—— but the last part was obliterated by the incoming rivulets of foam beginning to wash over it. The image was so striking, especially as I didn't know anybody by that name, that I wrote it down as soon as I woke up in case the significance might possibly reveal itself at a later date.

A year later, as the idea of writing this book was evolving in my mind, I went to see Alice, an old friend who has been associated for many years with the holistic health movement. I asked her to suggest some healers I could contact and courses I might apply to go on where I could learn more about how to develop my own emerging skills and get some practical advice. She gave me quite a lot of names from her address book and finally said, 'And there's a remarkable woman healer and aura reader by the name of Rosalyn Bruyere who runs the Healing Light Center in Glendale, California.' I had almost forgotten the dream until that moment and had to go home to check the name. There it was. I admit I felt a bit spooked, but also curiously excited, as if some plot were unfolding itself and I was a part of the drama. I wrote straight away to ask Rosalyn if we perhaps had known each other at school or if there was something else that could possibly explain why her name was in my mental filing cabinet, and whether, if I arranged to come to California, we would be able to meet.

I received an answer from her secretary saying that Rosalyn didn't recall that we had ever met as children even though we were about the same age, but yes, of course, I could come and visit the Healing Light Center. She enclosed a current brochure of courses available adding, 'Rosalyn will be giving a series of workshops in Ireland this summer if you're interested. Perhaps you'd rather come to those . . .'

What a bit of luck! Ireland! I've always wanted to go there. My mother was half Irish. I immediately booked up. Meanwhile I read a recent issue of the Healing Light Center's periodical *The Light Bearer*. It was all a bit excessive and embarrassing. One of the unfortunate aspects of the healing world is the tendency on the part of those involved in it to indulge in impenetrable jargon. There were advertisements for 'Certified Clearing Consultants' and 'Registered Rebirthers'. There were workshops to 'show the importance of physical reality as an integrated part of the total self'. You could send away for Audio Aura Correlation Tapes or book appointments with 'A highly skilled, loving and supportive fascillitator (Sic!)'. Dreadful Californian hype-speak. The articles were barely literate transcripts of taped lectures and the whole thing was distinctly resistible.

However, when the time came, I found myself crossing over on the ferry from Holyhead to Dublin, sitting up on deck in the hot summer sun reading George Trevelyan's *A Vision of the Aquarian Age*. Trevelyan believes the soul is undergoing a form of allegorical pilgrimage – a journey of the kind so often symbolized in classic myth – and he likens the body to a diving suit donned to protect the spirit from the immense pressures of the depths when exploring the ocean floor.

I hoped my suit would hold up when, scepticism fully operational, I arrived on the first morning at the hotel where the course was to be held. There were sixty other participants, mostly Irish, some English. The format was: teacher at the front with a blackboard and rows of chairs with the extroverts (me) bagging the front row and the quiet mice at the back. The size of the group seemed a bit unwieldy and after all my high hopes, I confess to feeling a bit disappointed to begin with, but gradually the nature of this section of my soul's pilgrimage began to reveal itself and by the end of the week I was quite intoxicated with the lessons I had learned.

Trevelyan speaks of 'those moments we are sometimes lucky enough to experience when everything appears fantastically beautiful and burgeoning with significance'. He believes these precious moments, once rare, are becoming more frequent as a universal tidal wave of consciousness swells up, gathering momentum and carrying with it a greater and greater number of surf-riders, hurtling skilfully on the foaming crest. I came home feeling that I was one of those crystal voyagers.

The first surprise was Rosalyn herself – sexy and flamboyant in six-inch turquoise stilettos and long dangly earrings – nothing like the homespun earnest puritan of my imagination. She was a dynamic, friendly, assertive woman, negotiating the trailing wires of her neck mike with all the practised flair of a rock star. Funny and warm; a bit too much glossy American hard-sell, perhaps, for British reticence, but a woman of strength and sincerity. I liked her immediately.

She began by telling us something about herself. She had a pretty rough childhood: 'Poor white trash on one side, lunatics on the other,' she said. She was dumped in an orphanage when her parents split up and raised by a great-grandmother who was psychic. When her great-grandfather died and the old lady carried on talking to him as if he was still there she was taken away, locked up and given electro-convulsive shock therapy. She never saw auras or heard voices again. 'But he was still there,' said Rosalyn.

She knew because she also had the gifts of clairvoyance and

clairaudience, but was terrified to use them in case they locked her up as well. She remembers seeing coloured lights around people as a small child, and knew in advance when family members were going to be ill. 'Most of us psychics are afraid we're crazy anyway because we don't get any validation of our experience from the outside world. There's nothing unique about me or what I do. People can be taught to see auras, to be healers and to let themselves get in touch with spirit guides. It's just a question of entertaining the possibility and taking responsibility for perceiving things for which there are no rational explanations.' She believes that all children are born with natural psychic abilities and are taught by ridicule not to believe in them. ('Stop making things up'; 'Don't tell whoppers'; 'Stop daydreaming and pay attention'.)

Rosalyn, lonely and isolated, longed to be a 'normal girl child' and suppressed her talents. It was only when she had children of her own that she knew she had a responsibility not to invalidate their experiences in the way that her own had been. Her kids babbled on about spirit playmates and fuzz around bodies and one day when her mother was visiting, the kids said, 'Why has granma got orange fuzz around her stomach?' Rosalyn looked and saw it too. Shortly after, granma was rushed to hospital with a bleeding ulcer. Rosalyn realized she had better stop denying her psychic abilities and begin to develop them. She attended classes in spirit communication, psychic perception and healing with a medium – she healed her own teacher of a nasty case of ulcerative colitis; her reputation spread and people began to beat a path to her door.

There are many psychics and clairvoyants working in the grey area of human distress. What makes Rosalyn different is her scientific curiosity. She studied engineering at university and loves to know how things work; she has consequently made herself available for a lot of laboratory testing and research work on the nature of the human aura.

She is now able to construct a teaching programme that integrates the science and the mysticism into a plausible whole. What she sees is a constantly changing luminous radiation of coloured lights surrounding the body. Disturbances show up as murky patches, enabling her quickly to diagnose the trouble and to treat it by channelling energy directly to where it's needed. She interprets the colours according to the chakra system. I was glad to hear her refer to something, at least, with which I had already become familiar.

The scientific research conducted at UCLA showed that there is a direct correspondence between the colours she sees and the wave patterns that show up on the oscilloscopes. Subjects being tested were undergoing a treatment known as Rolfing, a process of deep massage or manipulation designed to release trapped emotions and memories that keep the body tense and out of alignment. Electrodes were attached over their chakras to record the frequencies of the electro-magnetic field on a quarter of a million pounds' worth of hi-tech monitoring equipment. The correlation worked every time. Not all colour seers agree on what colours they see but Rosalyn's results are always consistent within her own frame of reference – and she works on the chakras because she feels that's the most efficient and simple way to get energy in and out of the body.

She believes that damage shows up in the aura three to six months before it manifests itself in the physical body. This aura, whatever it is – energy body; subtle, sensitive body – seems to react almost immediately to a shift of thought or mood or to changes in the environment. Some scientists think it may be a kind of plasma like streams of masses of ionized particles vibrating at different frequency rates. Right back in 1939, a Russian called Kirlian was attempting to develop a technique for photographing the aura. There is a continuing dispute about the accuracy of the interpretation of the results of Kirlian photography but one of the many startling revelations was that if you take a Kirlian photograph of a hand which has had a finger amputated – the aura will still show as a radiating outline where the finger used to be. This also happens if you cut away part of a leaf – the energy pattern of the whole leaf is still there: a sort of template for the whole. Modern exponents of Kirlian photography claim that, along with the electro-magnetic and thermal fields registered on the film, there is also a paranormal factor in the results which can give clues to a person's state of health.

Rosalyn thinks the aura is probably the mind, the governing intelligence in its wider aspect, and that it might eventually provide the long-awaited explanation needed to make sense of such phenomena as telepathy, out-of-body travel, and healing. Some interesting snippets of information arising from her fifteen years of work in this field are: that schizophrenics hardly have any aura but produce a three-and-a-half-foot plume of white light straight out of the top of their crown chakras. ('They are simply not at home,' she says. 'They are "out to lunch".') When a person has been meditating he or she has a blue-green aura which can also be achieved after aerobic exercise ('So if you can't meditate, don't worry, you can achieve the same contemplative state by jogging!'). Rosalyn can instantly spot drug abuse in kids' auras, which makes her an embarrassing guest at her own teenagers' parties, and she knows when someone is lying to her – their aura goes orangey-red.

At the end of the first day's lecture about the chakras and related mysteries, we tried some aura scanning on each other. First you rub your hands briskly together until you feel a sort of static electrical charge, the kind that picks up scraps of loo paper with a comb after you've run it through your hair. Then you scan your partner's auric space to see what kind of information you can receive. I was paired with a very short stout physiotherapist who works with handi-capped children. We made a hilarious couple and she had to stand on a chair to reach the top of my aura!

Altogether we were a very mixed group, with ages ranging from mid-twenties to late sixties and, for a change, nearly as many men as women. At this stage it was all a bit jokey. Although several people in the room were already practising healers, most were new to the game and quite reserved. I proved to be useless at seeing colours but it's certainly true that the confidence, subtle feelings, and seeings start to come more easily with practice. I could feel distinct temperature changes in a a person's auric field and I know more often now that I can effect a process by channelling energy.

'You're in an area where no one can validate you,' said Rosalyn. 'You have to learn to trust your feelings. If someone else feels it at the same time, that's data!' She recommends taking up a position of half-scientist, half-devotee. 'It's not just "Wow!" You need data as well as happenings.'

She told lots of anecdotes from her own experience to illustrate what she calls 'body symbology' – how the physical nature of the disease can often give you clues about the emotional and mental state that possibly contributed to it in the first place: lung disease can originate in a lack of freedom – literally not enough breathing space. Hypoglycaemia can be seen as a metaphor for 'not processing the sweetness in life', and kidney disease can mean you're 'pissed off'! In one case a man suffering from the alarmingly named ankylosing spondylitis (rheumatoid arthritis of the spine) was failing to respond to healing after many sessions. He was as rigid and stiff in his personality as he was becoming in his spine. One day she thought of asking him how he had allowed his thoughts to become so frozen, so calcified. He made the connection himself and began literally to unbend. The secret was to find out by enquiry, not by accusation. This experience taught Rosalyn two important lessons: firstly that anyone can be healed if they understand how they got ill. If they don't understand how they created the illness or the conditions in which it continues to flourish, and they won't take responsibility for it, they probably won't get better. Of course it's natural to express disillusionment and distress by blaming others, but growing up is owning your own luggage. And secondly not to give up on patients who are not healed spontaneously. Cases of cripples throwing away their crutches and running down the aisle are extremely rare. You are not a failure as a healer if the instantaneous cure is not forthcoming.

'This is not to diminish the miracle of spiritual healing,' said Rosalyn. 'The rest of the miracle is the taking of personal responsibility on the part of the patient, a commitment to change. A disease is of a damaged person, not just a damaged part. Also, don't be afraid to admit it if you're baffled. It makes the patient do the thinking which is often the key to their maintaining wellness.'

Rosalyn told the story of a friend she had healed of her chronic eczema after just one session, only to have her put on four stones in weight. All she had done was to displace the symptoms. People resist, she says, not because they don't want to be healed but because they don't want to be manipulated, and they cling to the familiarity of old patterns and roles because they are afraid of change. 'I'm not really into intervention,' she said. 'I prefer people to get on with their own process.' But she also likens the healing role to good parenting – being willing to take control at a certain stage. 'A good parent makes a child fit to live in the world. You have to be able to tell patients what they need, kindly, lovingly, comfortingly, and get them to move on before you both fall out of love. Healers have to work with push and pull. We have always been a very masculine-oriented culture – pushing and thrusting and literally ramming things down people's throats. What we need is a little more of the feminine principle: enfolding, drawing in, nourishing. If you are sensitive to what the patient needs they will take just the right amount. At the very least healing will provide a general tonic that re-charges the body's auto-immune system.'

She sent us away to do as much scanning homework as possible during the course of that first evening. Feeling rather cramped and stuffy after a day in the lecture room, I paired up with a man called Patrick – a printer from Dublin whom I'd briefly spoken to during the coffee break. We drove to a beautiful deserted sandy beach at Brittas Bay and had an invigorating but freezing swim in the Irish Sea followed by a jog along the shore. I found him a very easy, intelligent man to be with and within a short time we were discussing everything and anything with great candour as if we'd known each other for years.

Then we drove up to Amethyst where he was camping out and he shared his modest supper with me. Amethyst is a healing centre founded about three years ago by Alison Hunter. She trained with Rosalyn in California and is responsible for bringing her over here and publicizing the workshops. Regular courses, groups and private sessions are held here throughout the year by Alison herself as well as by a selection of visiting healers, lecturers and therapists.

Course participants who can't afford bed and breakfast accommodation in the town can bring their sleeping bags and sleep on the floor. It's a big open-plan attractively designed modern house in the foothills of the Wicklow mountains, with a communal kitchen in the middle. Very comfortable and not at all like a hostel – with superb views through the picture windows over the hills and surrounding countryside and away to the sea.

About ten people were staying there so there were plenty of guinea pigs for us all to try out our scanning homework. Strangely enough, for the first time ever, I could clearly make out an ectoplasmic sort of field around the person who was working on me – rather like the heat shimmer on hot asphalt. I can't really explain it, I certainly wasn't tired. Perhaps I am learning to see more intensely and the expanded awareness has begun to make my senses and perceptions more acute. There is always the nagging doubt that it may be self-delusion, wishful thinking, mind tricks – but if I didn't see it, what was it? When does the imagination become experience?

Patrick tried scanning my aura and said he could distinctly feel a lot of energy emanating from the higher chakras but a smaller, less dense field around the solar plexus. To put things in harmony he tried an energy-balancing healing on me, drawing up excess brow energy with his right hand and transmitting through his left hand into my abdomen. It felt very warm, relaxing and comforting, with slight erotic frissons. You can see how this sort of thing could quickly get out of hand. In fact all around the room people were enjoying hugs and quiet embraces. For many the experience of non-threatening physical contact imbued with a spirit of generosity was a new and remarkable experience. You actually feel the need to merge and express the big-heartedness and trust. Being sexually swept away would so easily and naturally follow on, but this is not quite a natural atmosphere – rather more like a space capsule – and in the real world of ties, bonds and responsibilities you might wake up to find you've created a complication with no happy ending. Everyone knew this. One of the great features of this work is the immense increase in self-awareness. You begin to understand 'where you are coming from', to use a useful Americanism, because you are forced to look at your own motivations.

I tried to feel Patrick's aura (a year ago I never would have believed I'd hear myself say that!). Like mine it seemed stronger at the top and weaker in the pelvic region so I balanced him up. Then I worked on a man called Jack with stiff tense shoulders and a pain in his groin. He reported instant improvement, which was very gratifying. And then Nora, with a bad hip and knee, who also experienced pain relief. Two men gave me healing for my lower back where I get tired aches, and it really helped. We all felt very powerful and pleased by the positive feedback. I am much more confident now about my channelling ability. I love doing this work and having contact with people at this essential and loving level. It really feels part of something beautiful and important.

This was also my first experience of Ireland and the Irish. The first revelation is how un-English it all is. It's at least as foreign as France, and the fact that we nearly speak the same language can be very misleading. Rosalyn's Californian colloquialisms create no end of open-mouthed mutual puzzlement. 'You guys don't know how to play!' she wailed in despair at one point. 'C'mon, gimme a break!' And she didn't know what to make of a timid question that began, 'I was after wondering . . .'

Patrick is a Catholic. As a young man he nearly became a priest but left the seminary after two years. I asked him about his views on the Catholic confession and absolution system in relation to healing. He explained that there's quite a revolution of thought going on here, where the idea of 'filling station' spirituality – drive in once a week with an empty tank and get it filled up – is recognized for the sham it is. You shouldn't just dump your wrong-doings and unload the responsibility; but rather use the confessional as a method for getting in touch with your deepest feelings about yourself as a human being. The priest, in the role of healer, should be skilful and wise enough to help you understand what you are doing, the patterns you create, and how you might want to change for the better.

Patrick is a rare light-filled person, small and slim with a great love of dancing. He dances as an expression of joy and is part of a liturgical dance group who perform on special occasions at Dublin Cathedral. He is also involved in leading a men's support group on a sort of mutual counselling basis and told me what an enormous pleasure it has been for him to be able to enjoy the company of other men in a non-competitive atmosphere of affection and trust. As a slightly built child and young man he learned to be very frightened of male aggression, and his upbringing made him alarmed and troubled by his own sexuality. In this group the men can talk, get angry, cry, hug each other, confide their insecurities and not be restricted by the awful conventions of pub machismo which force them to take up traditional male roles. 'Women's liberation has freed men to become vulnerable,' he said.

Everyone reported interesting results from their homework, but the question came up about the dangers to a healer of picking up other people's symptoms and feeling them in your own body. 'Healers are really warriors,' said Rosalyn (although she pronounced it 'woyers' and most people looked blank). 'That's not egotism – that's audacity. Preoccupation with self-protection is often based on paranoia.' The implication was that wimps need not apply. 'When you are feeling vulnerable, ground yourself and open more rather than trying to close down,' she urged, striding womanfully about, looking like Boadicea on the warpath. 'Once you're properly grounded you stop being a conduit for everyone else's rubbish.'

She gave us all a lesson in how to put our feet flat on the ground, toes uncurled, insteps pressed down. 'If you're channelling out you won't get symptoms,' she said, at the same time acknowledging that a certain amount of empathy is bound to be there. 'If you were totally immune you wouldn't understand what disease was, nor the patient's tremendous need to exorcise it.' This led to an interesting discussion about the rites of warriorship and the importance of understanding ritual and ceremony as a way of preparation and commitment to a life of service. 'There are times when people need a rite of passage to get them from one phase of development to the next,' she says, 'and healers need some kind of initiation ceremony which can take us from the position of ordinary citizens to that of magi, where a public commitment is made to serve as best you can.'

The native American Indians, of whom Rosalyn is an honorary medicine woman, have never lost these rites of passage and each step along the path is marked by various tests and magic ceremonies to enhance and underline the commitment to the next meaningful stage. Interestingly, you don't begin to be old enough to be a shaman until the age of sixty-five and you don't really become good at it until the age of eighty-one. Rosalyn is regarded by her Indian tribe as a rather precocious child – a baby healer.

The initiation rite for an Indian medicine man is a fearsome affair. He is given an infusion of peyote to drink which sweeps him away in a hurricane of frightening hallucinations: he is pushed off a precipice into the pit of Hell, there to wrestle with the devils of illness; he experiences all the pain and terror of their worst diseases until he eventually dies and rots. His bones are then gathered up in a pile and as he regains consciousness he experiences a feeling of being re-born with the knowledge of how to cure those diseases.

The symbolism is very interesting, implying, as Rosalyn says, that 'You probably have to have suffered in order to be a good healer.' But she added, 'There's nothing here that can hurt you. Come play!'

I loved her full frontal approach, her energy and her disarming vulgarity. ('I'm just a hooker for the Lord!' she said at one point, to gasps and nervous titters from some of the holier members of the audience.) But she was never offensive and was just as likely to drop in little jewels that shone with the pure incandescence of wisdom and truth. One of her most perceptive observations was that healers have to be able to deal with ambiguity and paradox. There is never one right answer and things aren't always as they seem.

We tried out some healing techniques for ourselves. One exercise was called, rather pretentiously I thought, brain balancing. However, it was not as alarming or dramatic as it sounded. It is done by placing the middle finger of each hand lightly just behind and above your patient's ears and channelling energy back and forth through the head. Someone suggested we could think of energy travelling like the wave movement of a shaken-out bed sheet. I found that helpful. The idea was to establish more of an equilibrium between the rational and intuitive hemispheres of the brain. In fact, this technique can be used with any part of the body. Apparently it's very effective with asthma and epilepsy. I certainly felt more alert after my partner had done me – as if I'd had a sort of spring clean and de-cobwebbing.

There is another technique Rosalyn calls 'chelation'. It is a general energy balancing of the body, starting at the feet and moving up through the joints and the chakras. It's a way of filling a patient up when he is depleted and it's often used as first aid when people are too sick to be treated. I found I needed a moment or two to attune myself to the person I was working with and to sense, with the aid of visualization, the energy running through my own body like a shimmering current of sparkling particles. Then as I laid my hands on my partner I felt able both to channel in and draw off energy, whichever seemed appropriate. I experienced a great tenderness towards my 'patient' and a sense of being guided by my higher self. The treatment took a long time and was very intense. Once you begin channelling, said Rosalyn, you are in a 'sacred space'. I think that is a beautiful description. There seems to be something hallowed about the transaction, where nothing is impossible. 'Be delicate with your movements, be reverent with the body,' she said. 'And remember, the patient is the best archaeologist on their dig. Ask them what they are feeling! Pay attention, listen for cues. Don't run your own trip.'

She also warned of the dangers of becoming what she calls a 'prima donna' healer – one of those who have trained themselves to work very self-indulgently. 'You know the type,' said Rosalyn. 'Gong, candle, incense, New Age tapes – give me a break! When you can no longer perform comforting without all the accoutrements, something is wrong.' A little humility from time to time wouldn't be a bad thing either. 'We all have the potential to help – I'm not sure we'll all be virtuosos. Born again, New

Age junkies beat everyone up with their "awareness". With the first flush of "Oh my God, my hands are magic!" people get really high, they get delusionary. They don't want to face the fact that they might not be the answer. Get out of the way. You're only there to help move the luggage.' A few of us squirmed a bit! Rosalyn is a wonderful sharpshooter.

On the chelation exercise I worked with Alison, the woman who is the inspiration behind Amethyst. A brave, resilient person – disabled by childhood polio but fiercely independent. She herself is a gifted healer and, because of her fortitude, greatly leaned on by other people. Of course, she is always hoping that it will be possible to restore the damaged motor nerves in her legs. Maybe one day.

Some people were getting a distinct feeling of heat from their healer's hands. 'Localized vasal dilation,' said Rosalyn, blinding everyone with science. And some people got rather emotional as their energies were moved about; there was quite a lot of crying and releasing as the group began to generate its magical safety net. Rosalyn observed that each group she works with creates an entirely different corporate energy. Ours, in her opinion, was predominantly serious, blocked, a bit sad, but loving and sincere, with a very high intelligence quotient. Since this was Ireland, the religious intensity was particularly palpable. Crises of faith, ecstatic transcendental love, repressed sexual conditioning, sublimation and explosive Celtic passions were lurking all around the room. Apart from Max, an ex-Anglican priest to whom I became quite close, there were at least three Jesuits and two nuns in mufti. A few people were depressed because they felt it was all over their heads and Rosalyn's style was too alien for them; a few were too needy themselves to be able to take in Rosalyn's most valuable and significant message: that the best way to be healed yourself is to heal others – it inevitably becomes a two-way process and you strengthen each other.

It's essential not to deny your own body's needs. Martyrdom and self-sacrifice do not necessarily equate with spirituality. As Rosalyn reminded us, 'It's hard to meditate when you're hungry, it's hard to love when you're angry, it's hard to share when

143

you're lonely.' Someone asked her about the condition known as 'psychic burn-out' suffered by some healers where they feel totally sapped and depleted. Rosalyn bristled with impatience. 'I get annoyed and bored by so-called psychic burn-out. It comes from being a martyr, giving out all the time but never allowing anything to come in, a refusal to be a part of the whole. If you take care of yourself and don't get hung up on rescue fantasies, it just won't happen.'

It was very encouraging to see how extraordinarily tactile everybody became as soon as they were given permission to touch each other and derive mutual pleasure from the experience, even in a largely restrained and sexually inhibited group such as ours – very blocked in this area of self-expression, but brimming with need and love.

We continued doing the chelating exercise with different partners for a whole afternoon and all felt considerably more balanced by the end of it.

Alas, Patrick was unable to stay for the whole of the course. He had to go back to work and was committed to his co-counselling group in the evenings but he offered to meet me up at Amethyst to give me a healing massage.

It was a beautiful gift, tender and generous. I felt very blissful and as cherished as a little baby. But I was not unaware that the feelings were more complicated than that. Patrick is a magical person, I am cheered by his ebullience. I admire his courage in being himself. He is articulate, demonstrative and married – and so am I. I suddenly saw how important it was to learn how to confront the sexual element which is inherent in the life force. It's obviously not appropriate to make love with every person you want to heal. But you can use those feelings in a transformational way.

Earlier, the issue had come up in a slightly different context. I was working with Max, the ex-Anglican priest – a sweet sad man, divorced from his wife, without his four children and recovering from recent surgery for bowel cancer. He was bravely trying to understand and alter the patterns of behaviour and response in his life that had got him into such a mess. He was only too aware of being terribly blocked in the area of his first chakra, symbolically speaking. His self-expression, his libido, and his *joie de vivre* have all been classically crushed by his childhood. He was worried that if he didn't get those energies moving, the cancer would return and get him somewhere else. He lives alone now with no outlet for his deeply passionate, inhibited nature and was feeling the lack of a partner in his life and in his bed.

How could I best help him? It made me think a lot about using this powerful, dangerous healing tool of sexual polarity. I knew that he was drawn to me and that I could assist him to have confidence in his own potency and his considerable qualities as a man – because I am a woman. But I was not the answer to his problems and my intervention would only be helpful in so far as I knew exactly what I was doing and what my reasons were. If my own motivation was muddled or if I sent signals that were in the slightest bit confusing then I would be harming not helping, destructive and dishonest. I wanted the woman in me to be able to heal the man in him without any strings attached. 'Intention' seemed to be the key word again. If my intentions were unequivocal I should be able to communicate without ambivalence, without capriciousness, the absolute sincerity in my heart. I was already aware of the dangerous tendency in myself towards what Rosalyn calls, with discomforting accuracy, the Great Western Tit syndrome! The desire to suckle the whole world. A lot of earth-mother-type women are prone to this one.

Max and I spent a day sightseeing together in Dublin. I confided to him my anxieties about not getting it right or giving him false expectations. It confirmed the wisdom that things are much better said than left unsaid. It cleared the air miraculously and left us both free to enjoy each other's company and walk about with arms companionably linked.

On the hills above Enniskerry, to the flaring accompaniment of a glorious Irish sunset, a social evening was held tonight for course participants to get to know one another. Patrick drove all the way there just for the party because he loves to dance and because he wanted to be with me. I felt very lucky to have found such a unique and passionate friend, but also conscious of the responsibility of keeping it all under control. The dancing was an exuberant free-for-all and we danced ourselves silly until 2 am.

I didn't know what was happening to me. I was buoyant and bouncy as if a hidden child in me had been set free – exploding with energy like how I remember being nine years old felt. Every day I got up at six and went running along the beach by myself in the morning. Some nights I only had four hours' sleep but as the sun rose I'd be bursting with vitality again. The other two ladies in my boarding-house were mildly disapproving. They were not enjoying the course very much; they felt they were floundering and it was all too dense, which proves you can't please everyone.

Rosalyn really got into her stride when we came to the subject on the agenda billed as 'Deepening the Healing Process'. Very intensive, practical and stimulating. I had to scribble furiously in my notebook to keep up with the flood of ideas. She gave further advice on how healers should look after themselves: take supplementary vitamins and minerals (counteracts a tendency to get too spaced out in meditation); avoid alcohol and sugar as much as possible ('fries the adrenal and makes your highs and lows violent'); drink at least eight glasses of water a day if you are doing a lot of channelling; exercise regularly (t'ai chi is one of the best types for healers – a good combination of meditation and balance); think of meditation not as a chore – something you have to *do* – but rather as contacting something you *are*. And if you do it better walking in the mountains don't waste time sitting cross-legged on the floor with the laundry list running through your brain. Keep a journal of your dreams and significant experiences to look back on.

She talked about the conditions which respond well to healing: diseases such as cancer, arthritis and cataracts react well, as the electrical charge from the healer's hands seems to stimulate the body's ability to reverse the degenerative process. Energy-balancing appears to be effective for such widely differing troubles as migraine and blocked Fallopian tubes. Rosalyn also claims success with cases of infertility. She says it's possible to reverse the negative and positive polarity of the ovaries where they don't match those of the woman's sexual partner. Patients with schizophrenia, fever, or high blood pressure can be helped by putting your hands on their heads and literally pushing them back into their bodies; inflammation can be reduced by drawing off excess energy and channelling a cool colour. Of course I haven't seen proof of any of this, but it ties in remarkably closely with what I saw Dr Kalii do in Kenya, so I have no reason to disbelieve. The important thing seems to be to work in co-operation rather than in competition with the medical profession.

We did lots of partnership exercises, holding hands and channelling energy round in a circle just to get the feel of it. Most people were a bit tentative. 'C'mon, beef it!' urged Rosalyn. I was feeling like a nuclear power station anyway and half expected smoke to come curling out of my ears. We tried an exercise in 'psychic duelling', where you deliberately try to block your partner's input. I remembered this one from my very first workshop with Andrew Watson and it's a killer. Rosalyn says this was an important part of a priest's twenty-eight-year-long training in the ancient Egyptian mystery school. Its value is in strengthening your partner by doing them the honour of being a worthy opponent – in giving them the opportunity to respond vigorously, to wrestle with the metaphorical dragons of energy and to zap through obstacles with knightly valiance. Your duty is to help your partner become the best warrior priest possible.

This was fun but exhausting. If ever one needed proof of the physical existence of psychic energy this, for me, irrefutably provides it. It's like pushing a car with the handbrake on. (My right arm continued to ache all the way up to the shoulder for five days.)

Rosalyn then showed us what she termed the 'healing wheel' technique, where you lay your patient on a table, place your hands underneath them and create a loop connecting your own body's energy field with theirs. You would use this method to channel out contaminated energy, discharging it harmlessly in the ground, when a person is too blocked even to receive healing.

She demonstrated on Tom, one of the Jesuits – a very fierce, gruff-looking man in his sixties. I'm sure it was not just coincidence that she picked him out of the group from where he was sitting at the back. His very posture and facial expression indicated the degree of tightness and disquiet in his body.

This was the first time I had actually seen Rosalyn work on anybody. She was extremely skilful and perceptive, picking up all his sense of sorrow, hopelessness and lack of self-esteem. She talked gently to him as she worked, her inner eyes seeing through the outer carapace to the great overflowing heartache there inside – an occupational hazard of a man with a lifetime of dealing with the pain and suffering of humanity. Suddenly, as she was channelling 'light into his heart', he began to weep, his body heaving and juddering with great sobs like old disused plumbing. He told her how unlovable he felt, how unworthy, while she continued to hold him and enfold him in a healing wheel of energy with her own body.

It was the most perfect and beautiful demonstration of using her femininity, her womanliness, her tenderness, to heal a tired and desiccated celibate old man. Watching her in action helped me to understand sexuality as a way of being in which the dual nature of mind and body is not in conflict but moves in harmony with the universe. She was a goddess, a priestess, as the web of golden light she spun surrounded him with compassion, filled up his heart with love, and discharged his pain. 'Did you ever think you'd see sixty pairs of eyes loving you?' she asked him and gently urged him to look around him. Many people in the group were moved to tears as they burned to comfort the old priest's despair. 'Allow some of that love to nourish you,' she encouraged. His dear old face lit up in a beatific smile and he returned to his seat profoundly changed.

Of course, this further underlined what, for me, had become the central theme of the whole week – how to come to terms with and transfigure the sensual element in spirituality. Rosalyn brought it up. 'I wonder why nobody's mentioned sex,' she said with refreshing directness. 'In most groups it comes up fairly early on!' She unquestionably has great sexual magnetism herself and has consequently been pondering the uses and misuses to which this can be put for some time. 'There is no such thing as a human exchange that is not sexual in nature,' she continued. 'Healers' energies don't become un-sexual but their attitude changes. Sexual energy becomes the life force and therefore sacred. You have to let that force keep moving up through you or you shrivel up. You can't deny it. It won't go away.

'The desire to merge with somebody else is very healthy,' she states simply. 'How else do I learn about maleness if I can't hold it in my arms? How else do I understand about other women's bodies? How do I comprehend "Warrior"? How does a man learn about "soft"?' As I am beginning to grasp it, true sexual maturity is a way of accepting and celebrating the energy of the life force as a power for good, a tool for healing. It is a commitment to this bodily incarnation with all its imperfections.

I guess this is what the much-misunderstood Hindu concept of the kundalini is all about. The fiery sexual energy, symbolized by a snake, rises from the base chakra and gradually becomes transformed as it moves up through all the centres to the crown where it vitalizes your enlightenment, so to speak. The very opposite of a licence for indiscriminate sexual experimentation, the liberating of the kundalini brings with it an awesome sense of sacredness and responsibility as it travels from the genital to the spiritual. The rising, twining twin snakes, one male, one female, around the staff of Apollo is still the symbol of the medical profession.

Rosalyn says that amongst the healers on her staff in California, some of the men have been outstandingly successful in curing breast cancer (Why? Because they love breasts and want them to be well) and women have been very effective at helping men with impotence problems. 'Try to think of yourself as a good lover in your patient/healer relationships,' she sums up with admirable clarity. 'Be tender, be considerate, ask "does that feel right?", give your very best.'

So what happens, I asked her, if you get a patient who doesn't understand the code, who hasn't heard of the life force and misinterprets your response as an invitation. 'Do you mean what happens when guys lust after you?' she laughed, sitting cross-legged on the table, looking gorgeous in black silk trousers and jewelled sandals. 'Now why would I know anything about that?' But then she added seriously that you have to convey to those patients who fall in love with you or think you are the missing ingredient in their lives that, although you are concerned about them and their problems, you are not the solution. 'Don't avoid the issue, though, don't pretend it isn't happening. Healers, therapists, doctors, analysts, all have to face this problem. When you are working with the needy there's always going to be the danger that they will fall in love with the first decent set of chakras that comes along – probably yours. Transference is a healthy process and enables the conscious mind to make a template for finding a finer mate – one with some of the qualities, perhaps, that the healer embodies.'

She told the story of her own experience of falling helplessly in love with her therapist a few years ago. He was not free and after the pain of coming to terms with the fantasy, she realized that what she really wanted was not him at all but a man with his qualities. She found one and is now happily married to Greg, a kind, strong, reassuring man who provides the perfect back-up support.

We worked for a long time on the healing wheel technique. Max gave me a whole hour of his devoted attention. I saw a lot of colours flood in great washes before my mind and felt a lot of energy moving. The kindness and the care are so restorative. It's only by being on the receiving end that one perceives how important that is. When I did him I became quite alarmed at just how blocked his body seemed to be, like a sewer full of sludge. I could hardly penetrate it, although I did manage to visualize catherine wheels of white light spinning at his first and second chakras. Curiously enough, just at that moment, his stomach began to rumble and gurgle and he said he felt a comforting warmth. So maybe something got through. I didn't feel happy about his state of health though.

On the fifth day of the course Rosalyn broached the important subject of the misuse of power. In America, apparently, there is a revival of interest in witchcraft associated with the extremist feminist movement which has tended to attract rather unstable disciples motivated by revenge and hatred of men for personal reasons – very unpleasant and manipulative. There is also a satanic movement which has claimed responsibility for ritual murders and other nasty occult practices. Perhaps even more dangerous are those so-called healers and mediums who have a very minimal understanding of the subject and who exploit and feed off those most desperately in need. A lot of that goes on.

Her message was to keep your wits about you, always be clear about the moral issues involved and look with self-awareness at your own processes. Self-discipline and a sense of humour should stop you getting too pompous or power mad. Beware the personality cult and traps of self-righteousness, she cautioned, but simultaneously be prepared to become one of the band of healer warriors who will stand up and fight for the human race. 'In our culture,' says Rosalyn, 'most of us, especially women, seek not to take power; we're too nice. Instead of training ourselves to handle it wisely, we leave it to those least suited to grab it all. It's important that we understand ritual and what ceremonial action is in order to prevent the Hitlers and other strong charismatic leaders from gaining control.'

All this was preparatory to the next stage of the workshop, 'Contacting Your Inner Guide'. Rosalyn has been practising mediumship for fifteen years and believes that, although healing is not something for which you need spiritual intervention, all of us have potential spirit guides and helpers if we only have ears to hear them. Guidance, according to the diagram she drew on the blackboard, is available on four different ascending levels. First and closest, on the astral level is our own personal 'gatekeeper', a sort of guardian angel often represented in symbolic form as a giant bird. At this level we often make contact with our first spirit guide, who might be a member of our own family. (Of course I remember my own initial tentative gropings in this area when I became aware of powerful feelings of being connected in a deep interior way to both my father and my mother's Auntie Violet. Nothing too alarming so far!)

At the next level, the etheric, we come across the 'teachers'.

These tend to be practical, matter-of-fact guides, often doctors themselves in a recent incarnation who still want to carry on using their knowledge and skills to heal patients. Rosalyn has a rough-diamond old country doctor from the California Gold Rush, named Dr Isaiah Johnson. At the celestial level are the 'master teachers', often from ancient civilizations – very wise and learned, with more profound spiritual advice to impart. Chinese philosophers, Egyptian priests and Indian chiefs come into this category. Rosalyn has a four-thousand-year-old Tibetan called Chi'ang. Should you be fortunate enough to have Jesus Himself, or the Holy Mother, or Mohammed or Moses, these are ketheric manifestations from the highest plane.

I have to admit I've had a lot of problems with this concept. I certainly don't want to rule it out – if there's one thing I've learned on my healing quest it is to allow for the possibility that anything can happen. Also, so many profound thinkers, mystics and poets that I admire and respect have no such doubts. I want to be neither gullible nor overly sceptical. I asked Rosalyn her views on the idea that the whole business of 'guidance' could be perceived in metaphorical terms – as something coming not from outside at all but from within. After all, the standard psychological explanation of what mediums do in a trance is that they are displaying their own alter egos. Rosalyn is fully aware of this rationalization but says that although some mediums appear to channel their own higher selves, to her, Chi'ang is absolutely an outside entity with a distinct cultural background and personality and an intelligence infinitely greater than her own. He is the one who has urged her to become a teacher, compelled her to spread the word, and continued to provide her with the vocabulary and flow of ideas without which she would not be equal to the task. 'Mediumship, like visualization, takes on a life of its own after a certain amount of practice. You don't want it to replace your intellect – only to blend with it,' she said. 'A questioning mind is important, but you don't want the part that says, "what if I made it all up?" to be too dominant.'

Members of the group with a strong religious background were quite nervous about opening themselves up to the possibility of possession by evil spirits. Rosalyn was adamant on this point. 'You only attract negative forces to the degree that you internally have an image of yourself as a victim, or when you are trying to obtain something you can't get any other way. It never happens to people who are genuinely seeking spiritual guidance.' But she warned that alcohol and drugs do not go well with mediumship. 'You have to be in total control of the experience. You're not seeking a manifestation as such, what you are trying to feel is something moving through you. Your own vibration bringing you into contact with the sacred.' You need to be alert and fully conscious but in an altered state.

The other warning was about self-indulgent style. Don't get into weird or theatrical behaviour and come on like a Madame Zaza-type fairground clairvoyant, straining your ears into the ether and intoning portentously, 'That answer comes to you from the Seventh Dimension', or insisting that you can only trance with freshly blooming lilacs in the room. Mediumship is a difficult and serious business and requires an internal discipline that most people can't be bothered with. 'Above all, don't scare yourself. A person needs comfort from their spiritual life, not stress. It's a way to grow up that you won't learn any other way,' she added interestingly. 'But if you don't feel comfortable with the idea, don't attempt it.' Her manner was wonderfully confident and breezy considering the enormity of the leap we were about to take. I felt like I did before my first jump when I once went on a parachuting course.

She explained the method for getting out of your body. You sit upright with eyes closed and concentrate on drawing your life force up through a wide core in the centre of your body, up through each chakra, and out in a plume of white light through the top of your head. You focus up into the white light, fly out above your body and look down on it. 'Plan your flight and fly your plan!' she teased in a joke aviation instructor's voice. We practised flying, first a few inches, then a bit more, and then several feet above the body. 'How can you see with your eyes closed?' asked somebody. 'How do you see in your dreams?' replied Rosalyn. 'Use the eyes in your astral body.' Simple!

As I understand it, this 'flight' is metaphorical but none the less real for that. If you experience flight, you are flying. I can only say I experienced flight. I felt my essence, wonderfully liberated and unfettered, drift on up to the ceiling and look back down on my body. We were supposed to notice if we could sense a presence or a shape of some kind. I couldn't sense anything other than a few other novice flyers bobbing about the room like Wendy, John and Michael from *Peter Pan*.

After we had returned to earth, Rosalyn said she could feel that Chi'ang, her guide, was around so she would leave and let him come in. She began to recite the Lord's Prayer, which is the method she uses to help her leave her body, and before she had finished, I witnessed an astonishing sight. Her body fleetingly took on the appearance of a person who has recently died – at that moment when you just know they've gone. Almost instantaneously I saw the most extraordinary manifestation of energy gather around her. It looked like a cloud of magnetic particles or a swarm of tiny black bees, resembling the radiating aura in a Kirlian photograph. She slumped a bit and as she sat up straight again her face took on a slightly thinner, masculine, oriental appearance. Her hand gestures and body movements became more Eastern and she began to speak in a rather hilarious Charlie Chan voice. All this could have been dismissed (as it afterwards was by several members of the group) as a bit of inspired acting or a corny con trick, but I have no reason to disbelieve. Why should she lie? I had trusted and respected everything else she'd said. Perhaps the strangest part and the most convincing was the very oriental style of the discourse, in the true tradition of sages and gurus who teach in riddles, set conundrums and leave you to figure out the meaning.

Everything she/he said was profound, mischievous, intelligent, and very different from Rosalyn's usual brash twentieth-century Californian personality. Chi'ang is rather fastidious, calm, wry and serene, although he doesn't suffer fools gladly. He admonished us for being such a humourless lot and finished his twenty-minute discourse with a few words of advice. 'Laughter and joy help the masters to come in,' he said. 'Do not take life too seriously, rather take it sincerely. Allow yourself to become more lovable. Become what you would love in others. No longer allow the darkness into the corners of your abode. Fill your life with lightness – in the food you eat, in your loving relationships and in play.' He left us with a Bônpo Tibetan prayer and Rosalyn opened her eyes.

Well, I don't know what happened – I only know what I experienced, and I am concerned that any attempt at explanation must do justice to it and should on no account devalue or interpret it away in order to fit it into a known frame of reference. I am increasingly aware that each individual must become his own authority, discover his own fundamental truth and be prepared to bear witness to it.

'Whether you are impressed by God, by guidance, or by your own higher self doesn't really matter,' says Rosalyn. 'If you experienced it, it happened.' When asked about the 'realness' of Chi'ang she said that he has defined himself thus: 'I don't exist in the way you think. I am energy just as you are energy. Until you realize the true nature of your existence you will not learn anything.' Another riddle.

Maybe there is a kinship that connects all human beings past and present into one great family. We do not fully understand the nature of time, and fragments of memory or experience from a different dimension sometimes surface out of context. Perhaps in the way we remember our dreams, we can learn to retrieve those snatches with more clarity and coherence, and to discover within ourselves several realities.

'Come on, play! Doesn't matter if you don't get it right!' cajoled Rosalyn, girding our loins for more flying lessons. I love the spirit of adventure and the promise of boundless horizons she brings to her work. We began with some super-sensitivity exercises exploring hand to hand touch, which created a highly charged tactile awareness. You were encouraged to see if you could sense your 'teacher' put a hand in yours while simultaneously feeling the great protective wings of your 'gatekeeper' about your shoulders. Without hesitation I had the comfortable sensation (memory?) of my father's right hand in mine. The shape of the fingers, the smoothness, the little scar, the slight indentation in the top of his index finger, the cornelian ring he always wore. I was half expecting it, so it came as a quiet joyous affirmation. Augmented, enabled, was what I felt.

The self-kidding aspect continued to nag me a bit but not as much. Perhaps it doesn't matter at what level it happens. After all, what are the criteria for judging something to be real? If I can experience the enhancement of my capabilities as positively as that, it's real. If it makes me stronger or more loving, gives me more courage or insight, it's valuable. Keats wrote: 'I am certain of nothing but the holiness of the heart's affections and the truth of imagination.'

The next exercise was to centre yourself, begin to run energy, open up to the possibility of guidance and allow your hand to move to where you could give a blessing to your partner. I was working with a small elderly white-haired woman. I touched her hand, she touched my shoulder. I wasn't aware of a 'guide', as such, but I did feel an increased capacity for love and output. I also felt a surge of energy coming into me from her so our little mutual blessing became a powerful reciprocal exchange.

The third exercise was to see if the guide would lead you to a particular needy area in your partner for healing. This time I did get a sense of being enfolded with energy around my arms like when someone is teaching you to play golf. Again the healing we did on each other felt augmented. The lesson for me, once more, was to expand the limitations of my current awareness and to listen to the inner voices of my own intuition. I still can't quite conceive of visitation from an outside entity but somehow creating symbolic mind pictures helped to bring extra power within my reach.

'I'm afraid of letting evil forces in,' said someone. 'Do you have any sense of what that evil may be?' replied Rosalyn. 'The devil, malevolence, madness . . .' people suggested. Rosalyn went on to say that in her opinion evil is indeed a very real force. It does exist, but its most dangerous and sinister form is the one that masquerades as good, eroding from the inside. The real dark forces among us were the warmongers, the Ayatollah Khomeinis;

the Rev. Paisleys; the American Fundamentalist Right; the police-state torturers; the propagators of hatred, fear and negativity. 'Pus pockets out of control, allowing the gangrene to set in.' Our own spiritual life should offer a measure of protection but, so saying, our first responsibility was to monitor the light and darkness in ourselves.

'You are going to serve where the devil works,' she said. 'You're right on the battlefield, so look to your own dark forces and try to clear them out.' That seemed pretty good advice to me. Self-awareness and the courage to stand against evil in the real world seem more important issues than worrying about malevolent spirits.

In the afternoon we had the pleasure of making the acquaintance of Dr Isaiah Johnson, Rosalyn's spirit teacher from the etheric level. I suspended my disbelief and enjoyed the experience. Rosalyn went into a trance and the good doctor came through with a hearty masculine voice (that slipped from time to time) and a slight stoop. I found it hard to take literally but undoubtedly something out of the ordinary was going on. Some people in the group could actually smell his pipe tobacco.

Dr Johnson is a very practical manifestation. He answered questions about specific clinical problems and gave some useful, if unorthodox, tips on good health maintenance. He told Max to flush out his colon with a coffee enema (!) – interesting in view of the fact that I'd confided to Rosalyn my worries about him; he recommended three drops of castor oil in your breakfast juice to protect your auto-immune system, oil your joints, help guard against AIDS and improve conditions of rheumatoid arthritis; he prescribed a quarter teaspoon of Epsom Salts in eight ounces of apple juice for spots, skin diseases, eczema and general cleansing of the liver; he suggested holding the colour turquoise over the thymus for allergies and hay fever; he said you should work on the feet for stomach disorders and he gave the recipe for a good cure for flu which could also be used as part of a regular diet – good for absorbing excess acid from the system – and to set the body up before a period of fasting. Here it is: one cup brown rice and half a cup of rye grains steamed in three cups of water.

After Dr Johnson had gone and Rosalyn returned to her normal self, she talked about ways in which small groups of friends could assist each other to explore the possibilities of mediumship. 'You don't all have to be mediums, but it is important that you all feel supported by the natural forces around you.' The gist was that to get beyond yourself and your earthly limitations you only need to embrace and welcome all the help you can get. You may not be the best healer in the world but there will be times when you are the only one there. 'It's an honour to be there when the miracle takes place,' she said.

At the end of the last day Chi'ang came through for a few last words. He said we were all interconnected in great bands of souls. 'When we help, serve, care for another we move closer to God.' He said the flow of the life force is a metaphor for the Path and that loving oneself is the honour we do to ourselves before God's love takes over. I asked him how it was possible to keep a sense of humour in the face of so much suffering in the world. 'If one sees only the tragedy instead of what is to come, existence would indeed be meaningless,' he answered. 'But when life and death is not the only issue, you can see beyond it and keep your sense of humour.' Other people asked a lot of questions to do with personal choices in their lives. The advice was kind and wise. Then he departed and Greg took Rosalyn home.

So that was it. Our little band of souls all hugged goodbye. Patrick came specially from Dublin to spend the last evening with me and a few of us climbed to the top of the sugarloaf mountain in the dramatic hills and rolling cloudscapes of the Wicklow Mountains. The sun, which hadn't appeared all day, suddenly came out for five minutes as we all stood together on the pinnacle with our arms around each other, feeling like giants, rejoicing in the holiness of the heart's affections and our new-found warrior-ship.

Later when we'd dropped the others off home, Patrick and I walked alone along the beach in the warm summer night and tried to sort out what it was we wanted from each other and come to terms with all that I had learned during the week about using sexual energy for healing. I absolutely adore him and I didn't want there to be anything that he expected or wanted from me that I wasn't prepared to give him. But a lover was not what I wanted. What I had already was far too precious to risk or dilute. I needed from him the freedom to be a child. I wanted to avoid getting drawn into the kind of heady escalating intimacy that leads to insoluble conflict and a bad ending. In return I gave him my precious crystal from around my neck because I wanted him to have something that was the very best of me, something much more intimate and binding than sex: a magic talisman, valuable and special, to convey the sacredness of the loving space we'd made for each other to grow in. We said goodbye, for the time being, and parted — the relationship to be continued by winged letters burning up the airspace over the Irish Sea.

Now comes the really strange part:

That night in the limbo land between sleeping and waking, I suddenly 'knew' with suffocating crushing horror, with anguished certainty, that Patrick and I had both been children together in a very recent incarnation and had died a violent and horrible death, snuffed out, bewildered, in the flower of innocence in a Nazi concentration camp. It entered my mind as a vivid subliminal flash like a scene lit up by lightning on a dark night — me with ratty pigtails, taller than him; both of us thin and raggedy, holding hands by a muddy trench. Palpitating, heart-stopping fear followed by blackness. That was all.

I sat up in bed profoundly shaken and pondered this revelation: it could explain a lot of puzzling aspects to this intense relationship. He frees me to feel very young and truthful. I have only known him for such a short time and yet, more than anyone I have ever met, he really sees me as I am and hears what I say. We can lark about with the artless daftness of kids, and there is also between us a grave childlike quality of reverence and awe. I do not want to be his mother or his therapist or his Great Western Tit. What I loved about him in the first place was his honesty and his courage to be himself - the very best man that he can be. He's freed himself to dance and play and not to be afraid. He's taught himself to choose life and to live it to the best of his ability.

159

I feel as if I've found him again, and that we can now finish our childhoods together and finally be allowed to grow up.

I guess that the whole episode is probably a symbol somewhere in the deep rivers of my psyche, a metaphor in my subconscious, for the omnipresent melancholy about the holocaust that infiltrated my childhood to a degree where unbearable feelings and unendurable realities had to be suppressed in order for life to go on. The knowledge of that horror and evil was always there at the back of my mind no matter how much I refused to face it, the burden of it somehow robbing me of the lighthearted innocence of childhood.

Only in Elisabeth Kübler-Ross's Life, Death and Transition workshop did the fact that all of that was such a deeply buried grief in me finally come to the surface. 'Why is your bird flying backwards?' Elisabeth had asked when she saw my spontaneous painting. The colour I had chosen, pale baby-blue, is associated with wholeness but also with death. The bird was flying back towards an uncompleted childhood where the tree I had drawn, although firmly rooted with a lot of vigorous growth, had very disconnected branches and no leaves. My childhood was loving and happy but very short – I married at seventeen.

Patrick nourishes me at a level that has always been hungry. He makes me become the best that I can be. Meeting him has triggered off some unfinished process. He is the childhood sweetheart I never finished knowing. Somewhere, in another dimension, I have known him and needed him all my life. 'I am certain of nothing but the holiness of the heart's affections and the truth of imagination.'

When Elisabeth Kübler-Ross was a young doctor she was part of the medical team that went into the infamous Majdanek concentration camp at the end of the war. Scratched on the walls of the children's quarters, in the midst of all that horror and suffering, they found drawings of butterflies – images of transformation and re-birth. She has used a butterfly ever since as her symbol for triumph over death.

My middle name is Imago. Only recently I discovered it means the final, fully developed state of a winged insect! Just to check, I looked it up in the *Penguin English Dictionary*. The other definition given was: 'Idealized memory or fantasy of a person beloved in one's childhood.'

6

Half the Understanding of the Answer is in the Question

After the visit to Dr John Muia Kalii in Kenya, I wrote an article about my experiences for a British women's magazine. During the following weeks I received a flood of correspondence, mostly from people in despair seeking a cure for some life-threatening illness and willing to try anything. But one long hand-written letter was different from the others and issued me with a challenge.

'Take this opportunity to come and see us. If you do not come now, you, along with the majority of the world's population, will certainly come in the future.' The writer was a Mrs Frances Vernon-Vaughan and the letter concerned her husband, Tony, a healer of extravagant claims who says he is the reincarnation of Jesus Christ. 'Before you dismiss us immediately out of hand as cranks, please try to keep an open mind! I do not expect you to believe me, only to accept that we are working for good and to try and improve the quality of life for everyone on Earth.'

She went on to describe Tony as 'a man with all the abilities you can imagine and those you cannot. He is logical, practical, and has complete knowledge of the Father and Heavenly Life. He is down-to-earth and totally aware of the past, present and future.' They call their organization the Pyramid Healers Trust and state their objectives, apart from giving healing, as being a training place for other healers, time travellers, past life readers, and telepathic guidance counsellors.

It was an offer I couldn't refuse. I was intrigued by the boldness and the battiness of the claim and the guileless tone of the letter. I answered saying I would be glad to accept their invitation. In the meantime I read some newspaper reports about the man. Mostly he is dismissed as a con man and a charlatan but there is a local Church of England vicar who has gone out on a limb to defend him.

'What impressed me', the Reverend Baycock is quoted as saying, 'is the fact that he makes no charge for healing and always makes it clear that his abilities come from God the Father. This indicates that he seeks nothing for himself.' He went on to ponder the question, 'How would people behave to Jesus if He came back today?' and concluded, 'Probably exactly as they did before and this is what is happening to Tony. People laugh at him and say he's barmy.

'Rejection is what Christians call the way of the cross. You do the right thing and people still say you are wrong. I think he's genuine. I have taken a lot of people to him for healing and they all say they have benefited.'

In his younger days Tony was a bit of a hobo, an odd-job man, driving lorries and emptying dustbins. Things went from bad to worse in his life and he began an inexorable downward slide until, finally, five years ago, he got kicked out of his rented bed-sit and became a ragged, dishevelled down-and-out, starving and shuffling through the streets of London.

One day, Good Friday in 1980, to be exact, he suffered a kind of fit. (As with Dr Kalii and others, a sudden episode like an electrical brainstorm seems to tweak the curtain of the universe and allow a direct brief glimpse of the infinite mysteries of existence.) He says he died then, but instead of that being the end, it was a new beginning. For four days he was locked in a straitjacket of total paralysis wherein he was taken on a journey of 20,000 years. In terrible agony he re-experienced the deaths of all his previous incarnations including, he says, the crucifixion, which is how he knows he was Jesus.

When he recovered on Easter Monday, he was no longer the same man, and he appears to have only a patchwork mosaic impression of that 'pre-death' time. He has been unromantically and uncharitably accused of being, in fact, the divorced father of six children and of having neglected his ageing mother, but he merely answers, unperturbed, that the man he once was is dead and he now is a healer.

His immodest assertion is that he knows and sees everything and everyone on the planet. That he understands every language there is or has ever been.

Apart from having been Jesus, he was also Moses, Elijah, Lao Tse Po, a 4,000-year-old Indian chief named Watering Cloud and Alexander the Great. I could hardly wait to see the man and gauge his claims for myself, so I travelled down to Kent to meet the Vernon-Vaughans.

Tony, over the past couple of years, has been training healers to disseminate the work and to leave him free for the bigger tasks, such as improving the quality of life. The Pyramid healers meet on Fridays and Saturdays in the front room of a bed and breakfast guest house called Abbey Lodge in Canterbury. I was greeted cordially by two of the women healers when I arrived. Gradually the place filled up with healers. They man the room continuously all day long until 10 pm, taking it in turns to go for meal breaks. Anyone can walk in off the street at any time. The service is entirely free – people are simply invited to place a donation in the box. The only rule is that you must specifically ask for healing if you want it, saying 'Will you heal me?' This formality preempts any charge that they are proselytizing or imposing anything on people against their will.

Unfortunately that day not a single customer turned up but nobody seemed deterred by that fact. They all did healing on each other instead. Every one of the healers first came here to be healed by Tony and they were all so changed by the experience that they now voluntarily come every week to pass on to others what they themselves received. Healers normally work in pairs. Once a patient has requested healing he or she is asked to sit comfortably with hands and feet uncrossed, 'to keep the channels open'. Then any two healers who are free at the time stand in front of the person about three feet away and say a short prayer.

'Our Father, I ask thee for the healing of this thine own child,

and I thank Thee in the name of the Father, Amen Amen Amen.'
Then for twenty minutes they radiate invisible laser beams of
energy from their hands like a benediction on to the patient.
There's nothing solemn about this and people chatter and joke
while it's going on. At the end of the healing, the healers draw
their hands together and kiss them in a gesture of thanks. That's
all there is to it. No physical contact at all.

The Vernon-Vaughans arrived mid-morning. Apparently Tony
doesn't put in a personal appearance very often these days
although he does take private appointments for a 'minimum
donation' of twenty pounds if anyone asks. However he came
today on my account and seemed willing to answer my questions.
There must have been twenty other healers in the room but
nobody else asked him anything. I felt a bit awkward being put
in the position of inquisitor with everyone else sitting around in
respectful silence, but in spite of repeated requests to the others
to enter into the dialogue, they all seemed happy just to listen
and learn from their beloved leader.

Tony is indeed a powerful charismatic presence. A tall well-
built man in his mid-forties, he still retains the weather-beaten
rugged look of a bloke who once lived rough. He has a kind,
faraway face with intense hypnotic blue eyes and bad teeth. He
stares a lot and laughs a lot, slapping his knee like a hillbilly. He
sometimes makes strange noises in a gibberish language as if
he's answering unseen voices, and occasionally describes weird
symbolic sign language in the air.

Some of the time he appeared perfectly normal, if a bit enigmatic, but most of his answers were evasive and cryptic as if he'd
learned them off by heart in advance. I asked him why some
people fail to respond to healing. 'On the first page of the Book
of Truth there is a mirror,' he answered. 'We begin the journey
to truth when we face the mirror.'

On death and dying he intoned, 'We are all like the leaf on the
tree that blows hither and thither, but it is inevitable that it shall
reach the ground and some leaves are nearer the ground than
others.'

I asked him why he talked in riddles instead of giving straight answers and I got this: 'My words are like the sun, my actions are like the moon, and the moon follows the sun. Sometimes the moon is obscured by cloud and you cannot see it but it is there.'

Occasionally his predictions were extremely specific: the conflict in Northern Ireland would be resolved in seventeen years, and (flattering music to my ears) this book would be quite good and would do well in Britain, Australia and particularly America where it would sell two copies for every one everywhere else! I had an important task to do in trying to communicate an awareness of healing – and of him – to the unawakened, he said, therefore I would be 'helped'.

Some predictions were pretty wild. How about this: within twenty years, the Pope (Tony reserves his greatest contempt for the Roman Catholic Church) would come to him seeking advice, and in order for His Holiness to be satisfied that Tony wasn't a charlatan, he would bring with him three children – one crippled, one deaf and dumb, and one blind – whom Tony would instantly heal. The Pope would, of course, be utterly convinced by this miracle and go home to Rome bearing the glad tidings.

No one would believe him, he would be sacked and banished and sent into the wilderness. Then one year later, on a calm still day, an unearthly wind would blow in the Vatican. A terrible ripping sound would be heard and the earth would open up in an orgy of biblical wrath to swallow up the entire Vatican. Just like that.

Tony told me he was planning to build a healing centre in the form of an enormous pyramid somewhere near Canterbury, and then another and then another. Within ten years, he says, the Pyramid Healers Trust will have grown to be the biggest organization of its kind ever known, with teams of reincarnation experts who are able to see your past lives; time travellers 'who help you actually to leave your body and find out for yourself about the past by witnessing it as it happened'; and others who can alter molecular structure.

The last capability will come in handy in his forthcoming confrontation with world leaders – before long they will have to listen to him, he says, and disarm, or he and his contingent of molecular reshufflers will crumble all metal to dust. Fortunately he forecasts that we will not destroy ourselves in a nuclear holocaust. 'Peace was promised and that promise shall be fulfilled,' says Tony. '"Thy will be done" means exactly what it says. It is not subject to human beings' belief or understanding.'

So, what to make of it all? In one sense it's laughable. Ridiculous. Superman in his pyramid-shaped Gotham City ready to spring into action and save the world – a childish fantasy. But then again, the trusting unworldliness of the man and his amiable nature make me ask myself, what harm does it do? As a philosophy of life it inhabits one of the wilder shores but it's no worse than some and better than many in that it involves its followers in optimistic, humane and philanthropic ideas.

Tony states emphatically that although he has all knowledge and all ability he has absolutely no personal power. He is merely a channel. All the power comes from the Father – he amplified that concept by saying that the Father is also the Mother, undifferentiated, unified, the Yin/Yang, the negative/positive, the Source. 'I'm not trying to convert anyone and I don't care if they believe me or not. The truth *is*, it does not attack and it does not defend. I base my work on love, kindness and gentleness. Anyone can heal.'

He talked very rapidly and I tried to remember some of the jumble of his remarks and predictions. 'Just wait and you will see that what I say is the truth and will come to pass. I never tell lies or flatter people and I am incapable of any negative thought or action. The world is full of negativity,' he said, 'created thus on purpose as a testing ground for human beings in this lifetime.'

'I have no desire for personal power or glory,' he said, 'only to be a mirror wherein the truth can be perceived.'

Much was made of the fact that life in a human form is extremely difficult for him. For example, he must never allow himself to get wet or he begins to 'short-circuit'. Although he is gaining strength and resilience he is still quite fragile and gets easily tired which is why he delegates a lot of the everyday healing work to his helpers.

Frances, his wife, is the perfect guardian of all these rare qualities. Very pretty and unquestioningly adoring and accepting, she caters to his rather bizarre physical needs and protects him from unsympathetic interrogation by answering some of the more aggressive questions herself. 'Tony is never wrong,' she interjected at one point. 'Not because he is clever, but because he is not allowed to be wrong. What he says may sound ludicrous, but it is backed up by his abilities. All this is done in order for people to accept the Father. Would the Father allow him to continue as he has for five years if he was lying?'

She also writes letters about him, spreads the word and has produced a baby daughter for him named Crystal. Frances is twenty-eight years old. She was married before to a man who ran off and left her with three small children. Managing the job of simultaneously shielding and publicizing Tony is now her life's work.

Tony looks very vulnerable – an easy target. I felt disinclined to quiz him about his life up until 1980, or to ask him, as many sceptical critics have done, to prove his claims about altering molecular structure or speaking ancient Phoenician, or what have you. It doesn't seem to matter, or rather it seems to miss the wider issues. He operates out of genuine love and compassion and although his claims sound almost comically boastful, there is a sort of simplicity and humility that stops you in your tracks and makes it seem unworthy and churlish to quibble over little details such as his throwaway line that he was once a prisoner of war in a Japanese camp.

He tells the story of another prisoner once risking a beating to give him courage by calling out 'God be with you!' as he was dragged away by guards, and of his answering, 'He will!' Forty years later in an English hospital, he came upon a man suffering from a serious life-threatening illness. He stopped to give him healing and as he went on his way said, 'God be with you!' 'He will!' whispered the man and in that instant they recognized each other with tears of joy.

Tony is not old enough to have been a Japanese prisoner of war – but then neither am I old enough to have been a nine-year-old child holding Patrick's hand in a German concentration camp . . . the layers of symbolic and collective experience we harbour have a validity nevertheless.

I asked Tony how he could illuminate the concept of reincarnation for me. As I understood his cryptic answer, it was that time and space are illusory. The Father is in all of us and we are all part of one another; therefore we have access at any time to experience an understanding in wider spheres. 'Before human life you were, and as it was in the beginning, so it shall be in the end,' he went on. 'The clouds gather and rain down on the earth forming streams which run into rivers, and the rivers run into oceans to evaporate and form clouds . . .'

Poetic facility isn't one of Tony's strongest gifts, but I remembered a quotation from Sholom Asch that I like very much. 'Our senses are haunted by fragmentary recollections of another life. They drift like torn clouds above the hills and valleys of the mind, and weave themselves into the incidents of our current existence . . .'

Tony had some unusual views on the subject of karma, the law of cause and effect. He believes that the karmic cycle is speeding up, rather like when you come to the end of a long-playing record. Whereas it used to take a lifetime before your ethical chickens came home to roost, soon it will take only three days. 'He who throws the stone shall be he who receives it. If you say bad things about me it will bounce back at you,' he warned, rather unsubtly, 'but if you help me, I will help you.' He smiled sweetly.

He offered to be at the end of a phone day or night if ever I needed advice or assistance with healing. I asked if it would be possible to affiliate myself to the Pyramid Healers and yet carry on healing using the methods I prefer, which involve more direct contact. It would not be possible, alas. In order to belong to their organization I would have to do it their way, in the name of the Father. He said the reason he teaches his particular form or 'manner' of healing is that, quite simply, it is the best way. It creates the purest channel and also removes the complication of sexual ambivalence in the healer/patient relationship. We agree to disagree. I guess I'll never be a joiner.

All his healers believe implicitly and literally everything he says, which always makes me uneasy. I remember Jim Jones, the screwy evangelist whose sect members did everything he told them, including committing mass suicide in Guyana by drinking Kool-Aid spiked with cyanide.

Tony concluded the audience by saying, 'My only wish is to open people's eyes to the power of love and kindness. Amazingly, some people find that a very unpopular message.' He embraced me and left.

I asked for healing on two separate occasions during the course of the weekend. I admitted that there wasn't anything wrong with me – I just wanted to experience the sensation. Firstly Sylvia, the chief healer, and Kate, who runs the boarding-house, combined forces. I must say it was an extraordinarily energizing phenomenon. My hands began to tingle first, then a general feeling of electrical charging, as if I was bathing in champagne, fizzed right the way through my body. An incipient headache I had disappeared and I felt extremely well. Later on the following day when Hazel and Patsy healed me, the effect was just the same – a great tonic.

The testimonies of the people here must also be taken seriously. The number of healers has grown in two years from seven to one hundred and twenty. Nearly everyone came initially for healing and received such profound life-changing benefits that they have become healers themselves. Anyone can do it easily, says Tony. You just have to ask to have yourself opened as a channel.

Patsy was born with severe curvature of the spine. A year ago she was 4' 11" tall. Today she is 5' 2", her spine has straightened considerably and the deformity is barely noticeable. More importantly she is confident, outgoing and attractive, where before she was self-conscious and introverted.

Len, a man with severe heart disease who was, in his words, a thorough sceptic, came here 'out of curiosity'. It's interesting how often sceptics just happen to find themselves in situations where they are proved wrong against their better judgement –

in other words, the preconditions for belief are already there although they're not aware of having created them. He was on a long waiting list for bypass surgery and didn't have much confidence in the consultant. Tony gave him some general healing and predicted that, through his psychic intercession, a bed would suddenly become available. Not only that – but a different surgeon, the leading expert in fact, would be brought in at the last moment. Everything came true exactly as foretold and Len is now a healer himself and a firm believer.

A woman crippled with arthritis, who was confined to a wheelchair and refused hip replacement surgery because she reacts badly to anaesthetics, was healed by Tony. She had first heard of him by reading a defamatory exposé of him in the *News of the World*. Nonetheless, she was mesmerized by the accompanying photograph and made her way here with her husband from Devon, a two-hundred-and-fifty-mile journey – convinced that this was the man for her. She is now walking well with the aid of a stick and her hands, which were all swollen, are perfectly flexible and normal. In fact, at the time of my visit, she had just finished knitting a boxful of doll's clothes for the Pyramid fund-raising fair.

Another woman I spoke to had suffered from lifelong asthma and hay fever – terrible panics about not being able to breathe made her whole life a frightening ordeal. Now she's cured, never had a single attack since her healing.

There are many quite young healers here too – eighteen- and nineteen-year-olds. Jamaican, English, Trinidadian, all races, all age-groups, all social classes. Young nurses, young lads, architects, solicitors, pensioners, unemployed people. I think one of the most effective aspects of treatment here is the ambience of reciprocity – giving healing is as important as receiving it.

Unquestionable is the spirit of jolly endeavour, the calm generous non-judgemental giving, the good humour and the articulate expression of belief in what they're doing. In the long run, gut feeling is the best barometer, and using mine, I would say that there is nothing sinister or hysterical going on here. The force is very positive and constructive – Tony appears to have tapped a great reservoir of dormant love energy that the Church, in its slumbering, has let slip through its fingers.

Tony states that his ultimate aim is to transcend the differences between religions. 'You go into a church hungry and you come out starving,' he says scornfully. He also criticizes the hypocrisy of churchgoers who don't back up their piety with action. 'You could pray a whole lifetime but it would not equal one act of kindness to a brother or sister.'

He has been given a hard time by the established church and is vociferously reviled by local churchmen, who call him a heretic and a blasphemer. They especially can't stand his claiming to be the reincarnation of Jesus. Because he doesn't conform to any recognizable norm, the establishment can't deal with him. He is an unknown quantity, therefore dangerous, therefore mad. True: people who hear voices can be either saints or sex-killers or mentally ill – ultimately you can only trust your intuition and the evidence of your eyes.

There are no easy answers to explain what's going on here. The claims made are so preposterous, so outrageous that even though Tony's disciples take them literally, I feel they can only be accepted in metaphorical terms – which isn't to diminish them in any way. The diminution comes more from the act of trying to capture a revelation in words, of trying to translate insight into everyday mundane language.

Tony's stories have a first-hand authenticity about them. There is an intensity and an immediacy in his perceived truths. He experienced all those things at some level of reality. The trouble is, once they become gospel – told and retold by unquestioning followers – they lose something. The real magnificence becomes moribund, embalmed in the fog of legend.

If you don't listen too literally to the words, but hear instead the higher message, it seems very clear – to me at least – that much goodness, kindness and unconditional love are flourishing in Canterbury.

Can one conceive, perhaps, of a life force, a collective force, as like an ocean of which individual human beings comprise the drops? Having come from the whole and remaining, even in our separateness, a part of the whole, we each contain, like a strand of DNA, all the coded information about the entirety – past, present and future. When we die, we don't remain as individuals and go off to join a crowd of souls in some vast celestial football stadium; instead we merge back into the oneness with Jesus, Buddha, Rembrandt, Mozart – any and everyone, including Chief Watering Cloud. The totality of human experience becomes available to us. We are the sum of all existence, and this is what we are tapping into when we have intimations of reincarnation.

In his simplicity and goodness of heart, Tony sees with the clarity of a new-born babe. In his face I see no intent to deceive, only the innocence of the Holy Fool and the clear gaze of a child. Who is to say that what he experiences as his reality is not the truth? I certainly wouldn't presume to judge him and I think that he himself is totally non-judgemental. All I can say is that the claims don't hurt anyone any more than Mohammed Ali saying 'I am the greatest' – so long as the power doesn't go to his head. If he's a con artist he'll get his comeuppance in time. Until then I feel it would be wrong to base an opinion on anything except his actions, which seem very Christian in the best sense of the word, as do his followers – unafraid to be thought mad or evil or possessed by the devil (all accusations which have been levelled at them); quietly getting on with it, giving their time and their love freely, accepting the brotherhood of man.

There are no conditions for joining other than an undertaking to give healing in the prescribed 'manner' and an acceptance of the Father, which can have a pretty wide interpretation. Anyone can become a healer; they only have to ask to be opened as a channel. Children under the age of sixteen who ask are made animal and plant healers. I loved that idea – so sweet and tender; encouraging the highest and most caring response, invaluable for the survival of our planet. Quite a few children are involved. One little boy told me solemnly how he had healed his dog after it had been scratched on the nose by a cat. Another said he was in charge of healing his mother's house plants. Children of the Aquarian Age.

There is another dimension to the healing here other than the purely physical and that is to do with improving the quality of life. I spoke to a Chinese woman healer whose elderly mother had died of cancer last year. She showed me a photograph of a serene old lady, laughing and animated, a few weeks before her death. Tony had been giving her healing and they all believe that although you cannot interfere with anyone's time span on this earth, you can do a lot towards helping to create peace of mind and a feeling of well-being. She died at home, surrounded by her family and friends, only drugged for pain at the very last – she was well prepared and eager for the journey. Her daughter saw it as a very successful death in spite of the grief to the family and the horrific nature of the cancer.

'Our healing is not based on faith. It is based on knowledge and understanding,' said Tony. 'And we never try to convince people to have healing against their will. You can only go halfway into a wood before you are coming out.'

Tony came into the guest house the following day to see a client who had requested a private consultation and he asked me if I'd like to sit in on the session to observe what goes on.

The young girl, Sue, was very nervous and overawed, like a small child in the presence of a department-store Father Christmas. She sat on the edge of the sofa with wild frizzly hair wearing endearingly ridiculous teenage fashions and clutching a prepared list of questions to ask him. Tony always works with two assistant healers, partly to protect himself against accusations of professional misconduct (insinuations to this effect have been made by the gentlemen of the press in their attacks on him) and also as a booster system.

He started by looking straight into Sue's eyes and saying gently, 'You've got yourself into quite a mess, haven't you?' This was a good move, implying tremendous clairvoyance on his part without committing him to anything definite.

Young Sue, feeling utterly transparent, burst into tears and asked for healing so the back-up team stood there beaming the rays at her while she blurted her questions out: Should she go back to Spain? Would Eduardo be waiting? Would her life straighten out? Would it take long? How could she give up drugs?

How could she be a better daughter to her parents and make it up to them for all the trouble she'd caused?

Tony answered cleverly and with great confidence, giving the impression that he knew everything about her but would only tell her what she was ready to hear. ('Half the understanding of the answer is in the question' was one of his more profound observations yesterday.)

She should take better care of herself for a start and not keep choosing the wrong men. Yes, she should go back to Spain, but within a week of arriving she would understand that it was not what she really wanted; there would be a couple of lovely relationships in store for her before she settled down; she should enjoy her youth but be careful not to get pregnant because, although single motherhood might be a valid choice for some women, it wasn't right for her.

He spoke sympathetically in simple direct language and with, above all, great self-assurance and authority – using the wise old wizard approach to great effect. Kindly but awe-inspiring he kept it lighthearted but grave enough not to devalue her problems. He promised immediate personal intervention in helping her to get off drugs. 'Wherever you are, whenever you're tempted, think of me, picture my face and ask for help – I will be there.' His eyes boggled at her hypnotically like a fairground Rasputin. He said that within three years her life would be sorted out.

The consultation lasted an hour. At the end she wept a lot and was hugged and comforted by one of the woman healers. 'Don't be ashamed of the tears,' said Tony. 'They are very healing.' It was a skilful and effective demonstration of picking up on the courage and hope a patient has displayed in taking the first step, and breathing life into the resolution to change. He had created an atmosphere, a space, wherein change was possible.

Later on I gave little Sue a lift back to London. During the two-hour trip she talked of nothing but how meeting Tony was the best thing that had ever happened to her. She was sure that this was the beginning of a whole new constructive phase of her life. No more drugs, repair relationship with parents, get her head together. I hope so. Certainly the new-found resolve will help to propel her quite a large part of the way. She asked me to drop her at the florist's shop near her house so she could buy her mum a bunch of flowers for the first time ever.

Earlier in the day when I had asked Tony how he would suggest I tackle an explanation of him and his work without alienating people not yet ready to hear his astonishing claims, he agreed it was a tough assignment to handle. 'The words will flow when you need to find them,' he said enigmatically. He conveys an unshakable certainty that the divine can be tapped at any time.

There's certainly much to be said for the quality of trust. Trust that if you are really trying to do your best and for the best of reasons, things that you need will come to you. The point is that once you activate in yourself the process of trust and back it up with affirmations, things start to happen in your favour and you begin to change old patterns. Whether you are trying to be creative or trying to reverse the process of a disease in your body, the same principles apply. Something more than mind over matter happens, something other than mere wishful thinking. It's as if the act of faith itself (whether in the power of your own 'higher self' or in an external force) is actually a trigger mechanism for the positive energy to start flowing.

'Only believe, and the belief creates the fact,' Dottie Snow pleaded back in Nashville when she was trying to get me to commit myself to Jesus. I think I'm beginning to understand the process.

The belief not only creates that-in-which-you-believe, but it releases the psychic power to move mountains — in some way it is the key which unlocks that part of the range of human abilities which transcends the confines of the logical, rational, intellectual mind, and bridges the chasm across into the realm of miracles.

Not that you necessarily have to become credulous, unquestioning sheep. The trick to learn is to be able to activate the process by a willing and conscious surrender to the unknown, and yet retain your own integrity.

It's an interesting fact that faith and humility, rather than great intellectual power, tend to be the characteristics generally associated with saints and healers, which seems to indicate that the intellect might be an actual hindrance. It constantly breathes in your ear, 'This can't be possible, this can't happen, this doesn't make sense.'

My mother was absolutely sure that when she died, she would be with my father again. It was such a positive conviction that there was no room for an alternative. Her faith was an abstract concept, of course, like love or hope – or rather a combination of both – but of such immense power that the energy it created would indeed have created the fact. Who can prove that she was deluded? No amount of cynicism or scepticism could have taken that certainty away from her.

Enough faith in something, with the aid of concentration, perhaps, or prayer or meditation, begins to create the conditions to bring about its attainment. The humility and the surrender constitute the act of plugging in, of linking up with the limitless reservoir of energy which flows from the source (inner or outer, depending on your belief system).

I've always resisted the term faith healing, because of the implication that a belief in God is a necessary precondition of the healing process. Although all healers, whatever their methods, share a common belief in the existence of a healing force that can be channelled through them to individuals in need, of course healing often works without any faith in it on the part of the patient (in the case of very young children, animals or mentally handicapped people, for example). Perhaps there's more 'trust' involved than focused 'faith'. What I've come to understand, I suppose, is that the abstract quality of faith in itself, as demonstrated by the placebo effect, hypnosis and autosuggestion, is a powerful tool for whatever you want to achieve.

It was in the early summer that I went to see Tony Vernon-Vaughan, and I gave much thought in the days that followed to the importance of the role a guru-figure can play in making you answer your own questions – being a staging post in the process of taking responsibility for your own life and your health. Then I met Norbu.

In the part of central Italy where I have spent my summers for the past fifteen years with my husband and children, we have a little house in a peaceful timeless medieval hill town. This summer, by astonishing and unlikely coincidence, a Tibetan lama, Namkhai Norbu, had come to southern Tuscany and established a community on the neighbouring mountain top.

Brendan, a young Irishman, had drifted in as a neophyte to orbit for a while in the light of the great one, and we got to know him when he applied for the job of builder's mate to help with some major structural repairs in our house that couldn't be postponed any longer.

Brendan was about six foot tall with a well-proportioned, well-formed body, lean and tanned from working as a labourer in the Italian summer sun. His scraggy ear-length hair looked as if it had been pruned with garden shears. On his head he wore a cheap builder's cap advertising a brand of cement. All his top teeth were missing, removed in childhood by an incompetent dentist and never subsequently replaced.

He wore a pair of baggy worn-out khaki trousers held up by a piece of string, a faded red T-shirt, battered second-hand shoes and a threadbare anorak. His only possession was a bicycle, on which he rode back and forth to Merigar, the Tibetan community, in the hills beyond the chestnut groves.

He turned out to be one of the most unusual and remarkable people I had met in a long time and I got a lot out of watching and learning from him. I feel certain it was no accident he happened to be here this year and I am intrigued by the phenomenon of synchronicity – seemingly random coincidences that connect bits of your life together.

To be 'aware' and to be 'present' were the basic tenets of Brendan's philosophy of life, and he would work willingly and good-humouredly, carrying buckets of cement all day long – never losing his temper or getting riled – all the while allowing his mind to turn inwards to ponder the deeper philosophical questions of the nature of man and the universe. He was interested and curious about everything, and derived profound satisfaction from the simplest of pleasures – the texture of hand-made brick or the smell of sardines grilling over a wood fire.

He is a potter by training and every so often goes home to his mother's house in Ireland to make some pots, grow some vegetables, bake bread and take stock. He has been on the road for years, a traveller without baggage, living with glass-blowers in Turkey, fishermen in Spain, and various other simple working people all over the world. The locals here had never encountered anyone like him before and after an initial period of open-mouthed amazement at his scarecrow appearance, have come to like and respect him for his friendliness and integrity. I frequently saw him sitting in the sun on a stone bench with some of the old men, or on the steps near the little piazza, energetically engaged in philosophical discourse in his fractured Italian!

He told me that the Dzogchen teaching of Namkhai Norbu that he follows has helped him find, primarily through meditation, a way to be 'mindful' in everything he does, and to be more aware – not only self-aware, but aware of the needs of others. I also learned that Norbu is a noted practitioner of Tibetan medicine, so I was very keen to make his acquaintance.

One evening after dark I went up with Brendan to Merigar to introduce myself and to pay my respects to the lama. In the village I had picked up a bit of gossip about the place and heard that curious locals were rather horrified by the general air of chaos and anarchy (although impressed by the large number of attractive female residents!). Certainly the dining-room looked a bit unappetizing – a great vat of spaghetti, a bucket of salad and gut-rot plonk – and slightly skiddy underfoot where the children had spilled their food. There was no electricity, just a couple of candles, and shadowy figures of unshaven aspect milled about in the darkness.

Norbu was being massaged by some loyal lady disciples in his private quarters when I arrived. It would have been inappropriate to barge in. A couple of others were cooking him a special dinner so I waited around talking to some of the community members. 'This is an unstructured environment,' explained a French resident with angelic-looking snotty-nosed children. 'You may, perhaps, find us a little bit too funky!' Because everyone is engaged in the pursuit of self-realization and self-determination, anything as authoritarian as a washing-up rota would be an intolerable restriction on personal liberty. Consequently it falls on the few who can't stand the squalor to clean up after everybody else. You could see these guilt gluttons slaving away in the gloom.

Merigar has a floating population of many nationalities, ranging from two or three hardy regulars who remain throughout the winter, to the twenty-five or so who are here now, to over three hundred short-stay visitors who came for the big retreat in August and camped in the surrounding hills (much to the consternation of the local constabulary, who muttered about inadequate sanitation and such). The place is being built piecemeal by their own labours and quite a lot has been accomplished already – a large communal meditation room, kitchen, dormitories, rudimentary ablution facilities, a Buddhist stupa – a little free-standing dome-shaped shrine that houses the sacred texts and relics – and the beginnings of a garden. The site itself is stupendous, chosen by Norbu because of its view across to a range of low hills that look, in sunset silhouette, like a sleeping pregnant woman.

Money for the building work and the regular running costs is raised by Norbu teaching and lecturing and auctioning, for exorbitant sums, the gifts he is constantly receiving from disciples.

Suddenly a whisper ran round the room that the master had finished having his massage and was now eating. I was told it was as good a time as any to make myself known. He was sitting with his Italian wife at a small wooden table in an upstairs room. Ranged along another at right angles to him were five or six disciples. According to Brendan, these are a self-selected group of courtiers who hang on his every word, laugh at his every joke, service his every need. Even when the air is thick with sycophancy, Norbu remains blithely ordinary, simple and accessible to all, but he does nothing to prevent the lionization and deification which is imposed on him by the needs of others. It's uncertain how much he actively encourages it but I suspect he doesn't have to at all.

I have been reading a book Brendan lent me, a verbatim transcript of some of Norbu's teachings. It makes heavy reading in translation but from what I have gleaned Dzogchen teaches that awareness, not only of self but of others, comes from the regular practice of meditation and non-attachment. The resulting clarity, truthfulness and state of being present produces a serene and non-judgemental attitude to the needs and actions of others.

The master, in his advanced stage of enlightenment, is obviously an adept at all this but from what I've heard, the principle of non-attachment creates quite a few misunderstandings for ordinary mortals who are inclined to interpret it as a licence to abandon any commitments, responsibilities or relationships which have become restricting and tedious. Many of those who come here with someone leave with someone else.

I can find no fault with the admirable simplicity of the teaching. It's always the wretched followers who mess things up by not being perfect.

Norbu himself is a man in his early fifties, stocky, strong and moon-faced, with thinning hair and sparse teeth. He has a rather endearing reputation for occasionally enjoying a jolly evening and a bottle or two of Brunello di Montalcino at the taverna in the town. Human and humorous by all accounts, he was dressed now in a red Italian designer tracksuit and seemed less than thrilled to be disturbed in the middle of his dinner, although he tolerated my presence.

I blurted out my mission, that I was a neighbour of his, that I was writing a book about healing, had heard he was a learned practitioner of Tibetan medicine and would love the opportunity to talk to him some time about the subject. He nodded and grunted but said nothing. I babbled on a bit more and then suggested that I perhaps come back at the weekend at a time convenient to him. He nodded again, we agreed on Saturday lunchtime, and I left him in peace.

All the acolytes looked rather stunned at my audacity – probably the correct procedure is to sit at his feet for several weeks in respectful reverence before speaking, but I guess sometimes it's an advantage to know nothing at all about a famous person because then one is not in awe of them.

When I got to Merigar on Saturday for our appointment,

Norbu and a few others were just finishing lunch in the glassed-in conservatory on the first floor. He had been watching me walk up the hill and was ready to receive me when I arrived. I greeted him this time in Italian and he was much more communicative. I restated my purpose in coming and he cordially invited me to sit down. He offered me fruit and wine but said nothing about healing. He had kindly found for me a pamphlet about the Institute of Tibetan Medicine in London and said I would be welcome to use their library to look up anything I wanted to know, but that was as far as conversation went.

He beamed, lay back with his eyes closed and had a little snooze. He was wearing dirty old clothes, his feet and fingernails were grimy, and he looked tired and dusty after his morning's work in the sun mixing cement. A young Italian disciple with a frail body and a drooping moustache tenderly took hold of one of the master's dirty feet, scooped a fingerful of home-made olive-oil, pine resin and beeswax pomade and massaged him as he slept. One by one, as they finished eating, people crept quietly in and sat themselves on the floor round the room.

I guess Norbu doesn't enter much into personal dialogues. His style is very much in the Eastern tradition where he imparts 'the Teaching' of 'the Practice' of Dzogchen and you learn what you're ready to hear. It's no use going to him with specific questions and expecting answers or advice about how to achieve enlightenment or sort out your life. He offers instead a mirror (as does Tony Vernon-Vaughan). You see what you're ready to have reflected and you understand what you're ready to know.

He has even written a little book called *The Mirror: Advice on Presence and Awareness*. In it he writes, 'If one neglects that which one has and instead seeks something else, one becomes like the beggar who had a precious stone for a pillow but not knowing it for what it was, had to go to such great pains to beg alms for a living.'

Although Norbu himself said nothing about healing, I heard from the others that he is very skilful in the Tibetan healing arts and has a wide knowledge of herbs and plants.

As I understand the basic principles of Tibetan medicine –

nothing in life can be separated from spiritual teaching and there is a clear relationship between mental processes and physical disorders. The causes of disease are classified under two main categories: immediate (infection, pestilence, climatic conditions and so on) and primordial (the original cause of all illness is ignorance of the true nature of being). So, in other words, unless you make some attempt at self-knowledge, you will be appallingly vulnerable to illness sneaking up on you at any time.

Tibetan medical practitioners develop their knowledge and gifts of clarity through the practice of meditation. Many of the great fundamental texts were written in the form of a dialogue between the individual and a state of original wisdom attained through contemplation.

Tibetan society also contained spiritual healers — lha-pas, or people of the Gods, shamanistic healers, and oracles deriving from the Bônpo tradition, who would go into trances and invoke deities. I had never heard of the Bônpo religion (the pre-Buddhist Tibetan religion) until Rosalyn Bruyere's workshop when she went into her Chi'ang routine. But here on a Tuscan mountain top only a couple of months later, I'm hearing about it again. The first medical teachings in Tibet originated from this ancient religious tradition which pre-dates Buddhism by several centuries.

Anyway, from our lack of spiritual awareness, come 'the Three Poisons': attachment, hatred and mental confusion. These, in turn, disturb the three finely tuned elements (perceived broadly as air, bile, and phlegm) and act upon the three interlinked components of human life: the body, the mind, and the voice (or vital energy).

The infinitely variable wrong combinations of these nine components produce between them just about any disease you could name. I was also interested to learn that the most important method of diagnosis used by Tibetan doctors is 'taking the pulse', a precise and complex skill that takes years to learn but is very similar, in essence, to Doc Kalii's technique of reading the blood in Africa.

There are also astrological considerations to be taken into account, similar to the Western concept of biorhythms — an individual's pattern of cycles, fixed from the moment of birth, which can be charted on a graph to establish 'critical' periods of vulnerability to illness.

Therapy is based on diet, fundamental lifestyle changes, the extensive pharmacopoeia of Tibetan medicine and external treatments such as massage. Also the chanting of a mantra (the use of a repeated sound at a particular vibrational frequency) is thought to have a beneficial effect and the power to act upon the body directly. There are links here with the way some New Age healers use colours, sounds and crystals in order to affect the chakras or energy centres in the body. The concept of using vibrational frequencies for healing has a long pedigree.

Finally, ritual, with symbols and musical instruments, may be employed to rally the body's defences and natural resources, but everything is ultimately down to the self-governing responsibility of the individual patient whose behaviour and attitude will be among the prime factors involved.

When Norbu was sufficiently refreshed from his nap he sat up and gave a little discourse on the subject of 'distractedness'. Everything is created by the mind, therefore maintaining a continuous state of mindfulness without allowing oneself to become distracted is very desirable. Most of us live very distractedly, allowing our energies to be dissipated by constant diversions. (It's significant that we use the expression 'presence of mind' to describe the condition of optimum effectiveness and quick response in a given situation.)

Beginning with the practice of meditation, one learns how to integrate awareness with all one's daily actions such as eating, walking, sleeping, working, and so on. Following the supreme path of continuous presence would lead eventually to a profound inner harmony and a state of bodily and mental well-being.

By now the master was in a very expansive mood. He told a couple of obscure jokes and people laughed like crazy. Then I listened while a woman named Louisa received a cryptic lesson involving the repetition several times of an Italian proverb about a fox and a rabbit. She obviously got a lot out of it and it clarified a point she was stuck on. Swooning with adoration and glowing with gratitude, she returned to the back of the room.

Later, when Norbu returned to his labours with the cement mixer, I got talking to Louisa – a very thoughtful woman of about my age. Originally American from a Jewish family, she has lived for many years in Holland and now speaks English with a Dutch accent. She has also travelled widely and lived in India for three years studying the sarangi with an Indian master. When she first set eyes on the instrument she knew she had a destiny with it.

I asked Louisa what it was she got from Norbu's teaching. She has been following him on and off for the past seven years. When she needs money she takes her sarangi to the main piazza in Grosseto and just sits there and plays. People like the music, she says, and find it peaceful and soothing. Norbu encouraged her to play when she had lost heart. By his example and his teaching she has begun to understand herself and to find 'clarity', a state she values above peace or tranquillity. She thinks he is a very great master and spoke interestingly on the relationship between guru and disciple.

The guru as mirror avoids simply revealing the truth. He uses images, parables, riddles and allegories to let people discover things for themselves. In the myths, religions and stories of every culture right back to the Stone Age, people needed gurus and shamans to help them on their spiritual journeys. The seeker comes in hope of finding someone to tell all the answers, explain the mysteries of the universe or cure him of his ills. Instead he finds a reflection of himself. ('What you see is what you get,' said Louisa.) Being able to accept that starting point with all its ambiguities and paradoxes is the beginning of change.

The way of the guru, for her, has been the best way. I don't think it would be my best way although I can see the value in it. It develops good habits like patience, stillness, humility and attentiveness. But it can also encourage lack of initiative, a slavish passivity and an unquestioning follow-my-leader mentality which sets up the right conditions for the Jim Jones scenario. The mindless baa-lamb potential of human beings and the spectre of mass hysteria always scares me but perhaps if you come at it from a position of awareness, or at least semi-awareness, you can make use of the best aspects and avoid the pitfalls.

Sheldon Kopp, in his brilliant book *If You See Buddha on the Road, Kill Him*, writes that ultimately, 'a grown-up can be no man's disciple. The most important things that each man must learn no one can teach him. Once he accepts this disappointment he will be able to stop depending on the therapist, the guru, who turns out to be just another struggling human being.'

Half the understanding of the answer is in the question.

Louisa offered to play for me. We sat on cushions on the wooden floor of the meditation room and she tuned her sarangi. It is a beautiful-looking instrument of elaborately carved wood, about the size of a fat viola. There are three main gut strings which are bowed and played by pressing up from underneath with the nails. Then there are dozens of tiny metal strings tuned to something like a scale of E♭ minor which resonate with sympathetic vibrations.

She played me one long improvised melody of magical heart-breaking beauty – a yearning, sweet, faraway sound; the sound of crystal mountains and sunlight in high altitudes. She closed her eyes and gave herself to the music, she became the music, and the room filled with the wistful longing. What wonderful meditation music it would be! Music to transport you beyond the boundaries of daily cares into the realm of communion.

As I listened I thought about the nature of this spiritual dimension and the words we use to try and describe it. Words like transcendent, cosmic, sublime are only inadequate approximations of this very simple state of surrender. Only when I am prepared to let go of the rigid structures of my everyday life do I release the boundaries and embrace the limitless possibilities. Rosalyn described it as a DC shift. It's almost as if a switch is thrown which then activates the other reality, the soul's reality, the state of union with other people and with the infinite – the healing mode.

All night long I kept thinking about this communion business and by one of those felicitous coincidences I got a chance to test and reinforce some of my ideas the following day.

It was a golden late September day and a celebration lunch had been arranged by friends amongst the resin-scented cicada-shrilling umbrella pines of the Mediterranean coast. The lunch was lovely – a real gutsy Italian feast and everyone stuffing their faces with sensuous appreciation. Roast pheasant, fresh vegetables from their garden, home-made pasta, fruit tart, and wine made from their own grapes. They were right in the middle of the *vendemmia*, the grape harvest, and one of the women, a certain vivacious merry widow named Natalina (the object of Brendan's attentions), was limping badly. She had injured her knee larking about in a tug-of-war while grape-picking and her leg was bound up in a bandage.

We were sitting around after lunch talking about healing. I asked if there were still, in the remoter rural areas of the region, people who practised traditional healing. I was told about a man who heals with magic water from a lake near his home in Massa Marittima. And there are apparently many old women still in the Amiata and Maremma region who cure people with herbs and roots and magic spells. There is a growing renewal of interest in these old wives' remedies here, as there is in England, and practitioners are beginning to come out of the closets where they were driven during the time of the great witchcraft paranoia.

I am usually a bit shy about offering, but on an impulse I heard myself saying to Natalina, 'Put your foot in my lap, I'm good at healing this kind of injury.' She looked apprehensive but I assured her I wouldn't do anything violent. I just put my hands on either side of her bad knee, visualized a cool, anti-inflammatory colour, a calming shade of blue, and channelled energy.

After about ten minutes, Natalina said she had a sensation like '*formiche*' (ants) in her toes. A great tingling current ran through her leg and there was a marked easing of the swelling and throbbing. Although we were both rather delighted, there was still a fair amount of pain and discomfort – Natalina asked if there was anything else I could try so I said I would send her some absent healing that evening and we made an appointment to focus our thoughts at 8 pm.

I confess that I've never had much faith in absent healing – never been quite able to understand how it worked. The physical contact seemed important to me in order to project the energy. Even working a few inches away from the body only seemed a kind of last resort if a person was in too much pain to be touched. But a mile away? Fifty miles away? The other side of the world? It seemed a bit far-fetched. However I said I'd try and I was encouraged by the strong bond we'd established of trust and confidence.

At eight o'clock we were still in the car driving home up into the mountains. I closed my eyes and placed my hands, palms up, on my thighs. I asked silently to be used as a channel for healing, and focused my concentration firmly on bringing Natalina's image to the centre of my mind's eye. I suddenly knew without any doubt at all that a part of what I call me was completely at liberty to traverse any space and find communion with the body I was seeking to heal.

Time and distance were no obstacle. The rush of energy was intense – immense. I felt like a fire hose. Without even trying, I visualized a rainbow pouring in through the top of my head and out through my hands to Natalina's leg. My hands were electric and the transmission of psychic energy quite unmistakable. I can only say that I was absolutely sure – I knew something had happened.

When I returned to ordinary reality in the front passenger seat, I told Richard what I had experienced and got the usual grilling I have to face every time this matter comes up as to the difference between what's 'actually real' and what's 'simply in the mind' or 'purely in the imagination'.

'The average person will never accept all that,' he says. 'It doesn't make sense. You have to bring the intellect to bear on this question, you have to use your critical faculties. When you say you leave your body, what do you mean? Can you travel down into the village and look through someone's window to see what they're having for dinner?'

I'm not really able yet to give a satisfactory explanation or a logical account. I ask myself, what leaves my body? What is left?

Where does the absent part go? What do I learn on the journey? The American writer Brugh Joy has said that we suffer from 'skin-bound consciousness' and that it is the mechanism of allowing rather than trying that enables us to make the quantum leap into a higher state of expanded consciousness. I think it's possible to be in two places at once just as it's possible to key into insights from a past life in some way. We are capable of so much more than we know. We can be here and we can be expanded, simultaneously.

There was a message waiting from Natalina when we got home, to ring her no matter how late. So I did. At exactly eight o'clock she had sat in a chair and concentrated her thoughts on healing, while trying to relax and surrender to the experience. Suddenly she felt an overwhelmingly powerful sensation of warmth and tingling in the bad leg and now, three hours later, both the pain and swelling were considerably reduced. She was amazed and excited and asked if I would do it again tomorrow. We arranged for 8 am and 8 pm.

The following morning I sat on the stone wall of my terrace to be in a quiet congenial place and to give my best attention to the healing. Exactly as the church clock struck eight, the sun moved from behind the tower and shone full on my face in a rather dramatic way, giving me a nice feeling of celestial intervention boosting the voltage.

Clocks were put back an hour last night to make this possible. All other days we'd been here the sun hadn't hit the terrace until nine. Once again I had the strongest feeling of contact and effectiveness. Without moving from the wall I flew across the landscape in the twinkling of an eye. I could be anywhere I wanted to be without crossing the space between.

However when the evening session was due, I was a bit distracted (sorry, Norbu). Although I concentrated quite hard, my mind was half on the fish I was cooking for dinner.

When Natalina phoned she was again delighted with the improvement from the morning's transmission but had forgotten to put her clock back and so had felt the effect an hour late. She also said, 'Did you forget this evening? I didn't feel anything.'

Nevertheless, the pain was gone. Her leg now felt well enough to walk on, and she returned to work the following day.

I still can't produce a rational explanation for what happened. Certainly, in spite of the time change anomaly and the fact that she could feel the difference when my concentration was diluted, autosuggestion on Natalina's part would have been an important contributory factor. But ultimately, I must have the courage of my convictions and say that it was more than that. I have opened the door to a much bigger room.

7

The Jewel in the Molasses

It was with these thoughts in mind that I staked all my publisher's advance on a round-the-world ticket. I wanted to go to the West Coast of America to do a course with Jack Schwartz at the Aletheia Psycho-Physical Foundation. I also wanted to visit the Australian Aborigines in the land of my birth, and I wanted to see the psychic healers in the Philippines.

I kept my plans pretty flexible to leave room for the governing principle I wanted to test: namely, that if you really trust your intuition you will always be in the right place at the right time. This is also a wonderful catch-all remedy for turning disasters into successes, for even if things don't turn out as you'd foreseen, you look instead for the lesson you're supposed to be learning and begin to see a pattern in everything.

The other important point is that no one else can be blamed. It's your responsibility whatever happens. It must be — energy picks up your signal and homes in on it. This is one of the central tenets of Jack Schwartz's teaching as I understand it, and it's also why I want to go and meet him: what you receive is a reflection of what you transmit — it's all to do with vibrational frequencies.

To be aware and to be present. Okay, I'll try, I'll try. It's no use perceiving all these truths and then not trying to live by them. 'Every pile of shit can also be seen as manure, it's a question of perception,' an analyst friend once pointed out to me. Growth out of dung, and all that. Whatever happened would be the story.

And it began with a whispering velvet flight in a Jumbo. I'm still a real kid in a plane. 'Start as you mean to go on,' I told myself, so I did what I've always wanted to do and asked if I could visit the flight deck as we were flying over such spectacular scenery: Iceland, Greenland, Baffin Island, Northern Canada and along the spine of the Rockies.

I chatted with the crew six miles up while we soared at five hundred and seventy miles an hour. Disconcertingly, nobody seemed to be actually flying the plane. 'Oh, don't worry,' said the captain, amused at my naivety, 'it's on automatic pilot. When we get to Mount Rainier, it will turn left.' It did. Very symbolic, and an excellent augury for things to come.

My oldest childhood friend, Sal, had taken time off to come up to Seattle to meet me and it was wonderful to see her again. Half dead from the long flight, I was swept up in the amazing excesses of the American style of life. Sal took me out to breakfast as the dawn light reflected magenta on the glass walls of gargantuan office blocks. It's quite common in the States to go out to breakfast and the Commerce Café had a staggering menu on offer of steak and hash-browns, pancakes with bacon and maple syrup, omelettes, muffins, French toast, fresh orange juice and unlimited coffee. The 'short stack' was six pancakes, each ten inches in diameter, and I didn't quite make it through to the end.

Sal lives in Longview, Washington, where for many years she worked as a saw-miller in the town's principal industry. It was a hard, dirty, dangerous job which she chose because it paid good money at a time when she needed to support her kids after her marriage broke up. A terrible accident in 1981 nearly severed her hand but the disability compensation she received enabled her to take the college degree she's always wanted.

We drove by the old house where she'd lived when she was rich and married, and looked down over the early morning Columbia River logging landscape that had dominated her existence for so long when she was poor and lonely. I was astounded by the transformation that had taken place in the five years since I last saw her – the confidence, radiance, and inner contentment that had come since she changed her life.

Now using her experience to work as a rehabilitation counsellor, and with a new loving partner in her life, she says that although she was never conscious of having cut her hand on

192

purpose, she is aware, looking back, of feeling that she would have done anything to escape. Even if she'd lost her whole hand it would have been worth it.

What prisons we build for ourselves! All she needed to do was leave, of course, but her spirit had to take such violent action to force the change upon her mind and body.

I had a couple of days in hand before Jack Schwartz's course, 'Tools and Skills for Transformation', so I picked up a copy of *Reflections*, Oregon State's quarterly resource directory, to see what was going on. What a feast! America at its hard-sell craziest. I wanted to try them all. Among the ads for tofu and T'ai chi were all the ways you could revamp your lifestyle or achieve instant enlightenment:

'A week's vacation in an hour? Experience floating in an isolation tank – a warm, enveloping, womb-like atmosphere in which to experience the beauty inside yourself again . . .'

'Catering is my art form . . . I can accommodate special diets and allergies . . . In your home I offer a hands-on class and/or dinner.'

There was an organization called Women With Heart Fighting Arts: '. . . emphasis on grabs, chokes, holds, blocks, strikes, and verbal confrontation.'

You could get a two-hour session with Jim, 'an exceptionally gifted psychic and metaphysical counsellor who will lovingly and powerfully guide you to a daily celebration of life and love'.

You could send for a current programme guide to KBOO.FM907, 'A non-profit community radio station which caters for black, Latino, disabled, Native American, and women's communities'. It also offered 'music tailored for women' ('Thank Heaven for Little Girls'?).

'Did you know: You can successfully love and live with more than one loving partner? . . . Find out more about Group Marriage from Polyfidelitous Educational Productions . . .'

This was the West Coast just as I'd always imagined it. I was really tempted by Jim, but in the end I plumped for this:

'Hello! We create a safe place for you to explore your own psychic space. We help you to get in touch with your own certainty. We teach you techniques that help you, as spirit, to understand the physical world around you, the ways of your body through which you manifest, and how to communicate with the God of your heart.'

The Church of Divine Man and the Washington Psychic Institute, founded by the Rt Rev. Doc. Slusher and his wife, the Rt Rev. Mary Ellen Flora, offer a one-year intensive seminary programme where anyone can become a Reverend. Also classes in body awareness, psychic meditation, spiritual healing and aura readings. I phoned up and spoke to a friendly woman, a graduate of the institute and an ordained minister. She explained to me how important it was to 'own your own space and to learn to see yourself as a spirit inhabiting a body. This is your moment, this is the time in the history of the universe for you to be effective.'

I couldn't argue with any of that, so I booked an appointment with Sheree for a 'female reading'.

Sal lent me her car, pointed out the scenic route to Portland, and I drove down on the Oregon side of the river, over Cornelius Pass, through the burnished October forests in the clear morning air. I got spectacularly lost in the tangle of interstate interchanges on the outskirts of Portland but eventually made it to the Church of Divine Man and felt ready for anything.

The institute was a comfortable old building looking rather like a private nursery school. On one wall was a chart with the names of the ten people in their current seminary programme. After each name were a number of merit stars. A big wall-hanging with 'HELLO' embroidered on it adorned another.

Sheree was a pretty, wholesome, fresh young woman with curly dark hair who sat me down and explained the format of the 'reading' to me. She produced a leaflet with matchstick bodies on it where she would fill in my 'programmability gauge', my 'male and female energies', my 'desire to bear children', my 'ownership of my body'. There was a space for her to draw a rose representing my present growth as a female.

She whipped out her receipt book and suggested we deal first with the little matter of the 'donation' of fifty dollars. 'Why the euphemism?' I asked, pointing out that if it was really a donation it would be considerably less than fifty dollars. She laughed merrily and muttered something about being a non-profit-making organization. Also, as I thought later, if you call it a donation, your clients can't claim they haven't had their money's worth.

We moved into the consulting room and sat facing each other on hard chairs with a tape recorder in between us. She said a little prayer to the supreme being – the God of our heart – then went on: 'Okay, hello there, Allegra! I'd like to begin by giving you a healing.' She closed her eyes and described a few strange patterns in the air with her hands. 'Do you mind if I move your mother out of your space?' she asked casually, 'she isn't leaving much room for you.'

And that pretty much set the tone of the whole thing. She had a fairly safe formula based on the premise that most women who come to her have a bad problem with their mothers (she herself obviously did, as I found out later when we were chatting). She harped on about my parents not letting me have my validation as a woman, about my not feeling at ease with my power, or fully inhabiting my 'female bardy'. 'Are you aware of working with your Mom's energy right now? Starting to clear out some of her concepts about being female which are different from yours?' She sighed deeply. 'I'm looking at a snake with two heads – the energy around that symbol has to do with fear about your power. I'm looking at a lot of your Mom's energy interfacing with you getting in touch with your own spiritual awareness. I'm seeing that having to do with your childhood a lot.'

('I don't accept that,' I interjected when I could get a word in edgeways. 'That's fine,' she smiled sweetly.)

'As a child you looked towards your father a lot to validate you in how you ran your female energy. But Dad didn't validate your energy, said no man would want you if you pushed your power.'

I felt she was way off beam on most things, inexperienced in areas of growth where I was considerably further along the path, and trying to impose a simplistic feminist stereotype on me with irritating cracker-barrel psychology. Along with the many things she got wrong, however, there was one interesting on-target hit:

'I'm looking at a lot of hidden sorrows that your father kept from you,' she said. 'Some of his dreams and fears affected you and there's a tendency for you to pull your father's grief in on yourself. You don't have to do that, it's not your problem.'

I thought she was missing the point. 'I choose to deal with that grief,' I answered. 'I'm neither unaware of it nor obsessed by it, but I think it's important to acknowledge it and understand it because it is part of me and I am part of him.' Sheree kept on smiling.

I got 46% on the 'programmability gauge', although it was never made clear what that meant. And there was a lot of bright green creative energy flowing up from my reproductive centre and out through the crown chakra signifying my desire to bear children.

At the end of the session I made my points of dissension. 'That's okay,' she smiled, 'you're entitled to your opinion.'

It was sad to see how this lop-sided over-simplified perspective of woman as total victim has often become standard formula thinking in the feminist movement, and how the sexes are much more polarized in America than in England.

'This whole women's programme is designed to help females recognize their unique bodies, the energies we have to use and how to re-own them. A lot of women really have a problem with that,' said Sheree afterwards. 'That's why I took the two-year training.'

I agree there is a need for that but many women most in need of 'validation' are the very ones who can least afford a donation of fifty dollars. There is also a danger of a built-in warp in a programme designed with so many preconceived ideas. Surely men have just as many difficulties getting 'validation' as children, for the more feminine side of their natures. 'Owning your own space' is something we all need to do, but it's a comparatively recent notion and most parents of anyone over forty bumbled along, doing their best within the framework of the values of the time.

Forgiveness for the inevitable mistakes seems to me to be the way to move forward rather than this constant bitching and blaming that goes on all the time. I guess what saddened me was the lack of real insight or wisdom. Sheree was still grinding her own axe. An expensive lesson for me but a useful reminder that there are plenty of non-starters and blind alleys on the healing trail, I reflected as I drove back to Longview along the freeway in the evening light.

I confess that before I arrived here I was slightly unsure of what my feelings would be staying in a lesbian household. But any awkwardness on my part instantly evaporated in the warmth of Sal and Josie's loving home. They each have a teenage daughter living with them and, of course, it's just a family of people like any other.

As we lay around on the floor listening to music and trying to cram the years into a few hours, I gave Sal some healing for her damaged hand. She has all kinds of hardware in there and her doctors have told her she'll never get the usage of it back because of excessive scar tissue. They have made a brilliant job of stitching her back together again but it seems a shame to be so negative about the prognosis. I can't see why it shouldn't be possible to stimulate new tissue growth by regular channelling of life-force energy and by visualizing the condition improving.

Rosalyn Bruyere told the story of a severe burn case she was called in to treat because the patient's body kept rejecting the skin grafts. The surgeons tried once more and Rosalyn came every day to give him healing. There was great optimism about the experiment, and when the big day came to remove the dressings they were all horrified as the skin graft came away again – *but underneath the patient's own skin had completely grown back without any scarring.* We still don't understand how the power of consciousness can affect energy and matter but there seems to be enough evidence around to make it worth trying.

I showed Josie how she could help Sal by talking her into a state of deep relaxation, getting her mind into a positive mode by thinking of something happy or inspirational, focusing that feeling of well-being on to the damaged hand and visualizing it beginning to loosen, become more flexible and strengthen. Even seeing it as completely whole again, playing tennis, making pottery – but above all having faith in the body's remarkable healing powers. During the visualization process, Josie could just channel energy straight into the hand.

Sal said she felt tingling in her little finger where she had felt no sensation at all since the accident so we were all rather pleased with ourselves and felt quite excited by the possibilities.

They offered to drive me all the way to Ashland, where my course was taking place on the Californian border, just so that we could all spend a little bit more time together. A real gesture of friendship indeed, as it would be a long eight-hour slog, and I was grateful for the company.

The roadside neon billboards along the freeway would make a great subject for a photographic essay. I especially enjoyed the one advertising the 'DRIVE-IN CHRISTIAN FAMILY CENTER: KARATE, BIBLE STUDY, EXORCISM, SELF-DEFENSE . . .'

We stayed the night with Sal's sister along the way and in the morning drove on into Ashland to look for Jack Schwartz's brand-new establishment, the Aletheia HEART (Health Education and Research Trust) Center just moved here from Grant's Pass. It had only recently opened and ours was to be the first course held in the new buildings.

My heart sank a bit when I saw it. The place is right on the main highway – a very nondescript, unpromising-looking building in the middle of a car park, with no garden; not at all like the architect's drawing on the brochure. No one was there at 9 am and the doors were locked. The course was meant to begin at 10 am and I had travelled over six thousand miles to be here.

It was one of those moments – the first of many on this trip – when a frisson of doubt appeared to mar my cosmic plan. 'Oh God! This is going to be disaster,' runs the internal dialogue. 'Relax! What happened to being in the right place at the right time?' 'But there's nobody here. It's probably been cancelled. The organization's gone bust. I'm going to be alone in the middle of

Oregon. I don't have any transport. I've wasted my money. My onward flight leaves from San Francisco . . .' 'Worry is a useless waste of energy. Whatever happens is the story, remember?'

My chums were reluctant to abandon me on the doorstep so we sat in the car park to give it a bit longer. Just before 10 am, I was astonished and delighted to see my friend Alice appear. I had received a postcard from her, sent from California, just before I left London, saying she was toying with the idea of doing the workshop just for the hell of it and because I was going to be there. I never seriously thought she'd make it but I should have known better – she is mistress of the unfettered, spontaneous gesture. More than anyone I know, she finds some way of going where she feels she ought to be at any given moment. It was she who had first suggested Rosalyn Bruyere's name, along with those of a selection of other healers from her address book, right back at the beginning of this adventure.

Alice is a counsellor, healer, teacher, actress, theatre director and inspired tarot reader – a catalyst in many people's lives, a candle flame at which others light their tapers. But she has paid a high price for these qualities. At fifty years old, she has no home, no children, no permanent relationship, but earns her living where she can and travels the world seeking and learning and sharing her wisdom.

I was so pleased to see her and offered a red-faced apology to the cosmos for my faint-heartedness! What was more, she'd booked into the excellent local youth hostel where there was a spare bed for me, and she'd rented a little car so we could drive to San Francisco together when the course had finished. Everything fell into place brilliantly; Josie and Sal drove off relieved, Aletheia opened its doors and the Tools and Skills workshop was under way.

'This is not a course in obedience. It is a course in disobedience. Disobedience to me – obedience only to your higher self,' began Jack Schwartz. This was a good opening gambit considering my recent musings on the nature and purpose of gurus.

Jack Schwartz, a Dutch yogi, is one of the great characters of the New Age movement. He has been around the West Coast scene since the hippy sixties, with their encounter groups and the first stirrings of interest in serious paranormal research.

As a child in Holland he became aware of his clairvoyant powers and healing abilities early on. When he was nine years old, his bed-ridden mother began to feel a lessening of the pain where he touched her, and within three months she was out of bed and able to move around for the first time in years. He became the neighbourhood boy wonder and people would arrive with sick relatives and animals for him to cure.

His hands seemed to be magnetically drawn to the right spots. He perceived emanations of coloured light surrounding the body and, noticing that the colours changed when his hands entered that auric space, began to realize he was dealing with some kind of energy field.

As he grew up he became fascinated by the mind's ability to override the body's so-called involuntary processes. If yogis could do it, why couldn't he? He taught himself to perform several amazing feats such as lying on beds of nails and walking on hot coals. His exuberance and natural sense of showmanship led him into a career as a stage hypnotist and cabaret fakir. His death-defying act was in great demand, he was beginning to get quite a name for himself and to set his sights on fame and riches, when the Second World War engulfed Holland and altered, forever, the course of his life. He joined the Dutch Resistance and was captured by the Nazis.

Events that destroy some people can be the making of others. Jack's experiences in the concentration camp taught him the lessons that he has tried to live by for all his life since.

'I saw that those who emerged with bitterness only looked at what they had lost, not what they had learned,' he said. 'They were consumed with hatred and the desire for revenge. What I gained was insight into myself. I recognized the true meaning of freedom and I found a higher purpose in life – to demonstrate to the world that hatred can never prevail over the power of love.'

The energy we radiate is crucial in determining the energy we attract to ourselves. As you transmit, so shall you receive. The principle of resonance underlines his whole approach to healing.

Jack Schwartz is a tall thin man in his sixties with abundant wiry grey hair, and a thin wiry grey moustache. His face is open and friendly with laughing crow's-feet and an unforced, spontaneous, happy expression. He is a Tigger sort of person — bouncy and boundless. He uses his whole body all the time, springing about the lecture room, leaning across the tables, leaping up and down. His enthusiasm is very infectious, if a bit exhausting — like a wire-haired terrier dragging you along at the other end of the leash. Sometimes I longed for him to stand still for a minute.

Constantly firing questions at his audience to make sure we were on the ball, zooming off at every tangent — the one really hard thing for him to do was to stick to the syllabus. 'Tools and Skills For Transformation' became 'How to survive a weekend with fuel-injected, turbo-charged Jack Schwartz.'

'What is the substance of the universe?' he demanded, sticking his face one inch from mine. ('Um, Er!') 'Energy! The universe is energy. We are individualized energy. What am I? I am human energy. The trouble is that most of our belief systems dam up and stagnate our natural life-energy, and this contraction of energy, this holding in, is what causes physiological problems.'

For the past twenty years Jack has been actively involved with scientific research programmes into self-healing and voluntary control of the body. In a famous series of filmed experiments at the Menninger Foundation in Topeka, Kansas, he demonstrated he could shove knitting needles through his biceps with no bleeding and no pain, causing the wounds to heal within hours of the needle being withdrawn.

'My whole life's work has been to show people that these potentials exist and that only self-imposed restraints prevent us from tapping into them for self-healing and for greater mind-body harmony,' he says.

Being willing to take risks figured high on his list of priorities. 'Risking is a tool. The prime tool of your life,' he said. 'Excitement and enthusiasm are two others. Take the leap of faith. Say "Yes" to life. Abandon yourself to the unknown. The only place where the divine will can be found is within the seat of your own consciousness. It takes a lot of courage to enter the unknown realms of the inner self.

'Trust your own authority. Dare to follow your own sensitivity to know when and what and where. Don't elevate others' opinions above your own inner knowing. Jesus said, "Ye can do the things I do and greater things will ye do." You can learn techniques, but don't get stuck in them — we've got enough technicians in this world already.'

This was why I liked him so much — that great big-hearted zest, that quality of curiosity; wanting to see round the next corner, over the next hill, down the next rabbit-hole. His risking is another way of describing my surrender — a state of vitality without the defences that normally keep life at a safe distance.

'My intuition never fails me, but I fail when I fail to listen to my intuition,' he said.

Breathing techniques are at the heart of all Jack's teaching. The theory is that different breathing patterns cause a change in the brain waves, enabling you to control and regulate such processes as heart rate, blood volume, temperature and pain reflexes. 'But why stop there?' he reasoned; 'Can't we also influence malignant growths, infection, the regeneration of tissue and bone?' He has done hundreds of his self-inflicted wound demonstrations and never uses a sterilized needle.

The implications are enormous and Jack's work at the Menninger greatly contributed to the development of biofeedback techniques. Now with the help of self-monitoring equipment (essentially electrodes on the scalp attached to meters that measure electrical activity in the brain), subjects can get instant feedback about what's going on. This is of immense value to patients with high blood pressure, for example; if a bodily event can be associated with a recognizable mental state then it should be possible to control the bodily event. This has led to teaching self-control through self-awareness and arriving at an acceptable theory of the interaction between mind and body.

'I realized that every time I went into an altered state of

consciousness, my breathing pattern changed,' said Jack. 'Prana, ki, chi, light, the life force, whatever you call it, breathing is the key to expanded capabilities. If you never do anything else, study proper breathing.'

He warned us not slavishly to imitate oriental breathing techniques, however, because our physiology is significantly different. 'Use it as a springboard, a template, but do it your way. Adapt it to our environment.'

Drawing on the work of Maxwell Cade and doctors Elmer and Alyce Green who pioneered the experiments, Jack defines the four brain-wave rhythms as follows:

Beta rhythm at a frequency of 13-30 cycles per second. This is the normal waking rhythm associated with active, questioning linear thinking and concrete problem-solving. It is a shallow, upper chest breathing with a high-frequency, low-amplitude wave.

Alpha rhythm at a frequency of 8-13 cycles per second. This is a relaxed, passive rhythm associated with inwardly directed attention, meditation and feelings of contentment, like a cat when it's purring. It is abdominal breathing with some diaphragmatic expansion.

Theta rhythm at a frequency of 4-7 cycles per second. This frequency appears in dreaming, daydreaming and visualizations. It is lower abdominal breathing and is associated with access to the unconscious mind, deep meditation and creative inspiration.

Delta rhythm at ½-4 cycles per second. Low-frequency, high-amplitude diaphragmatic breathing is associated with deep sleep and, paradoxically, with higher levels of consciousness and paranormal phenomena.

There is even a minus delta, but I think you may be one degree above dead then, or certainly in a coma. This is the one yogis use when they get themselves buried alive or incarcerated in stone sarcophagi.

'If you are resonating purely on beta you will receive only

local stations,' says Jack. 'Whereas theta waves reach beyond restrictions of time and space. Like a logo on a balloon, consciousness expands with breathing.'

He is good at providing colourful imagery and physiological explanations for the chemical changes that take place in the body when you alter the brain-wave pattern by exhaling over a longer count. Things like oxygen and glucose content in the blood alter dramatically.

We practised gradually extending the outbreath with this exercise:

Breathe in for four counts
Hold for four
Breathe out for four
Pause for four
Repeat three times

Then each subsequent time we were to try and lengthen the outbreath, to eight counts, then sixteen, then thirty-two.

Thirty-two was impossible for everyone the first time we tried it but after a few attempts, most of us could even manage sixty-four. With each extension of the outbreath, you encourage the theta state – the transpersonal state – opening doors into bigger rooms leading into still bigger rooms. Such a tremendous feeling of adventure, all these endless realms of possibilities just there for the taking. 'Theta breathing physiologically blocks out lesser energy,' says Jack. 'It keeps negativity at bay.'

Sitting there in a horseshoe formation with a dozen other heavy breathers practising our next assignment, Tibetan eye-rolling, I reflected on how much I have changed this year. I have grown and I have flown and I have learned a thousand new things. Will I find the words to share this sense of discovery and fun? Am I managing to keep my sanity? My sense of humour? My feet on the ground? My credibility? I don't want to lose sight of my starting point but it has receded so quickly into the distance. Like the Apollo launching pad, the charred debris of my former support structure has fallen by the wayside as the mysteries of the universe beckon me further out.

'The state of not having to defend oneself against the truth of one's own being is relaxation itself,' says Jack, bouncing about the room. 'A state which allows a person to conserve great amounts of energy.'

What this means in practical terms, in Jack's case, is that he only needs an average of two hours' sleep a night, he says. His wife, Lois, is a delightful contrast to him. A lady of generous proportions and serene aspect, she has obviously found a way to balance his perpetual motion. Jack also claims to eat only three meals a week and has a plausible theory about how it is possible to get all the nutrients we need from the sun. It goes something like this: since like attracts like, if we radiate out a certain frequency of energy, we attract from the environment a particle of the same frequency. He works up such a state of high energy that he practically glows with celestial incandescence. He processes undiluted cosmic energy in the form of sunlight and mainlines it straight into his pineal gland, thus bypassing all the middlemen in the food chain.

It would certainly be a handy accomplishment in times of famine but it seemed a bit advanced for my current stage of development. Anyway, I enjoy food (and I would guess Lois does as well).

During the lunch break Alice and I indulged in the earthly pleasures of a delicious asparagus quiche at a local health-food joint. Jack came and sat at our table for a few minutes. He beamed his psychic aura-reading powers on me and said some marvellously encouraging things: that my role in the greater scheme of things was to be as a harmonious blender, a creative artist who would use my gifts to clarify and demystify some of this esoteric stuff for people to read. 'I can hardly wait to see your book,' he said, 'because it will be truthful and innocent. You have the gift of remaining forever childlike.'

He was also very interested in my amethyst ring – the large, carved Mexican face set in silver that I always wear. The ring used to belong to my mother and she gave it to me just before she died, along with a wonderful story about its history – that it was a magical amulet obtained for her by my father from an extremely powerful Mexican shaman. It's such a good story that I've simply ignored the distinct possibility that it may have been purchased in the Portobello Road. I love it very much and I've always felt, long before I even heard about the healing properties of crystals, that it was special in some way – a transformer, an amplifier. Now here was Jack saying that it had the ability to capture and distil all the energy in its range of frequencies for me to draw on. The purple ray. The ray of transformation!

In the afternoon he enlarged on this concept of rays. In addition to emanating energy in the form of an aura or etheric body, he says, we each have an incoming ray – a vortex-shaped input current. As the aura reflects, in a glow around your body, the sum total of your past experiences, your state of health, your spiritual development, so the ray shows your potential.

Jack endeavoured to explain his perception. He sees the ray as a conical shaft of pure white light beaming down into each individual. As it comes in contact with the prism of the human aura, it refracts into different colours. The aura then absorbs all the sympathetic frequencies leaving only the colour of the energy frequency that you are seeking to actualize in this lifetime. Therefore, knowing the colour of your incoming ray can give you an important insight into your purpose in being alive. It shows what you are capable of. It illuminates the tools in your toolbox.

Jack uses the ray as a powerful tool in diagnosis and counselling. It gives him useful clues as to areas where a patient is not utilizing or fulfilling their potential. 'The ray is the main power line, the main current of energy to the individual from the universe,' he says. 'The pure white light that will be distributed throughout the body by means of the chakra system. The predominant colour that shows up represents the most important qualities an individual has to work with.'

There are seven different rays. Just for the record, they are:

| FIRST RAY: | *Colours:* | red, white and electric blue. |
| | *Qualities:* | power, will, courage, leadership, self-reliance. |

SECOND RAY:	Colours:	azure blue and golden yellow.
	Qualities:	love, wisdom, insight, intuition.
THIRD RAY:	Colour:	emerald green.
	Qualities:	comprehension, mental power, adaptability, tact, impartiality.
FOURTH RAY:	Colour:	tawny bronze orange.
	Qualities:	stability, harmony, rhythm, beauty, balance.
FIFTH RAY:	Colour:	lemon yellow.
	Qualities:	logic, accuracy, tolerance, patience.
SIXTH RAY:	Colour:	rose pink.
	Qualities:	one-pointedness, devotion, sacrificial love, loyalty.
SEVENTH RAY:	Colour:	purple.
	Qualities:	precision, grace, dignity, nobility, activity, integration, ritualism, designing, synthesizing, transforming.

This is all slightly complicated by the fact that some people may have combination rays. You also have to bear in mind that everyone has all the qualities in varying degrees but we each have a unique mixture.

Jack's own ray, he says, is seventy per cent pink on the inside and thirty per cent blue on the outside, which he interprets as the pink ray of service to others tempered by the blue of will-power and cool authority.

Mine is the fourth ray, he told me, the tawny bronze orange one. In his book *Human Energy Systems*, he goes into all the rays in detail. I looked mine up. It's not all good news. Along with being able to bask in the harmony and beauty aspects, people on my ray have to beware of a tendency to 'become cosmic sponges, psychically absorbing everything around them whether it's positive or negative'. We also 'like to be in the middle of everything, even to the point of meddling in other people's problems'. And worse still: 'they become so eager to fulfil their ray that they try to bring harmony everywhere. At times they will use any method to attract the attention and involvement of other people so that they can play a controlling role in life.'

I'd better take heed. A cross between Shirley Temple and Rebecca of Sunnybrook Farm. (I also remembered another pearl of wisdom from my analyst friend – the same one who gave me the advice about making compost from life's excrement. 'The compulsion to give all the time is very controlling,' she cautioned. 'It's a preemptive shot. You're buying insurance. Don't be too mean to be needy.')

I think one of Jack's main points here is gently to remind any would-be healers to be aware of their own motivation before presuming to engage in someone else's healing process – to be able to distinguish their own problems from those of the person they're trying to help. It's interesting to note, too, how we will take criticism when it's couched in these tactful terms. If he'd merely told me that I was an interfering old busybody who believed everything anyone told her, I would have resisted it – denied it. But the fact that my ray showed up those tendencies . . .

It's not necessary to be clairvoyant in order to see rays and auras. Anyone can train and develop their sensitivity by practising Jack's special eye exercises, also detailed in the book. Like the tarot, or Bruce MacManaway's dowsing pendulum, aura reading seems to me to be a way of fine-tuning your intuitive insights, augmenting your senses, sharpening your awareness.

A final caution from Jack is to take it all with a grain of salt. It isn't definitive or infallible and ultimately each person is the best judge of what is applicable to them. 'If you can give the fruits of your vision to others,' says he, 'and encourage them to keep what is valuable and throw out the rest, then you have truly been of service to them.'

Alice and I had a whole dormitory to ourselves as it was the low season. The youth hostel is a paragon of good design and good organization, and all for four dollars a night. To ensure the smooth running of the place, everyone is expected to pick a chore from a list on the board and you sign your name against it when you've done it.

I woke up early and went for a magical, invigorating run in Ashland's Lithia Park beside the stream and through the fallen copper leaves of the frosty autumn morning. Then I swept the front porch of the hostel and had breakfast with Alice in a cosy café.

One essential piece of advice I can pass on to workshop groupies and seekers of wisdom and truth is the absolute necessity of engaging in some form of bracing physical exercise before spending the rest of the day sitting on your bum. You can get a bit spiritually top-heavy if you're not careful. Now feeling charged with oxygen I was ready to take on part two of this course.

Jack Schwartz has a very individual, idiosyncratic teaching style. Part ham actor, part mad professor – but he really knows his stuff anatomically and always tries to relate the mystical theory to the practical usage. We began with the point raised yesterday about risk. It is, he says, allowing a continuous state of excitement, arousal and reciprocity. Taking energy from the universe and returning it. It's not that you don't question things, but rather that you shouldn't let yourself get hung up waiting for an answer.

'Just put your question out into orbit – don't always be seeking confirmation of what you know. Trust that you know it. If you constantly hold on to questions, you are working from a contracted, low-amplitude beta brain wave which is not the healing mode. Forget healing from afar, you can't even work from close.'

This is what I discovered for myself in Italy, the day of Natalina's absent healing – that if you wholeheartedly try for a state of humbleness and trust, you may feel appallingly vulnerable but you are, in fact, much more powerful. You are immediately in touch with the 'satellite stations' rather than the 'local agricultural news', as Jack puts it.

If you keep waiting for answers instead of taking a risk on your intuition, if you forever hover indecisively, you get 'cold feet' both figuratively and literally. You store charged blood in your head instead of letting it go and, consequently, are susceptible to poor circulation and migraine. One of the biofeedback techniques developed at the Menninger trains people to divert excessive blood flow from the cerebral area back to the peripheral parts of the circulatory system, making the head cool and the hands and feet warm.

I like the way Jack constantly stresses the importance of understanding the psycho-physiological processes. 'We're here to demystify your body,' he says. 'Forget metaphysics until you understand what's actually happening in the body. All visions, insights, metaphysical psi-isms and premonitions can be nicely explained within physical laws. Which means you don't have to be a special saintly person to have them – just in physical, emotional and mental control.'

Since most of us aren't anywhere near being in physical, emotional and mental control, we spend most of the day trying to get in the driving seat.

The dance of energy seems to be the basic law of life whether you approach it from the viewpoint of particle physics or divine essence. Jack's current hypothesis, which makes sense to me, is that we human beings process energy and transform it from light to fire via the chakra system. To demystify these mysteries and make them accessible, Jack tries to give practical physiological explanations for things. For example, in much the same way that we take in breath via the lungs, utilize what we need, and expel the rest, so we also take in, via the pineal gland and down through the metaphysical chakra system, the subtle substance of pure light from which we extract nourishment and fuel before returning it to the ether. Jack makes it clear that he is making symbolic statements about the body in his attempts to communicate what he 'sees' – subtle, non-visible, non-physical forces and multi-dimensional planes of consciousness – phenomena which have not been verified in scientific laboratories but which nonetheless are clearly visible to him.

The chakras can be thought of as little dynamos, he says, closely interrelated with the endocrine glands, regulating and distributing the energy along the spinal column – each one resonating to a different colour, sound and vibrational frequency – maintaining the organism in harmonious balance. Therefore an unimpeded flow of energy is the key to well-being. When a chakra's function gets dammed up and the flow becomes sluggish or restricted in some way, either from a physical or an emotional cause, the energy is not being transformed and it stagnates.

'Stagnant pools become cess-pools,' says Jack, 'full of gases, toxins and poisons.' In other words the energy becomes denser and duller. Our immunity factor deteriorates and we begin to attract toxic substances and low, negative vibrations because we are resonating at a level which is electromagnetically sympathetic to all the rubbish in the universe. We are literally calling the stuff in on ourselves. Setting ourselves up as victims.

'Making molasses,' is his metaphor for this proclivity of ours. Drawing all your energy in like a snail's horns, condensing it, letting your light dim, as you disappear up your own black hole.

I could understand what he was getting at and it was exactly what I was ready to hear: Risk it! Come to grips with the anxiety of the possibility of loss, even of non-being. If you really let yourself go with it, with the willingness to change and grow, you will expand and unfurl and then there are no limits to what might come your way – maybe even miracles. Fear limits our ability to live freely. 'All diseases are labelled fear of change,' says Jack, 'and the biggest fear is the fear of fear.'

Anyway, the point is that in order to maintain equanimity in the face of life's vicissitudes, you have to start radiating outwards. Jack calls this 'finding the jewel in the molasses'. To be going on with, we learned a simple exercise for clearing your own spine of energy blockages. Place one hand on your crown chakra and the other on your tail bone. In most people, the left hand is the negative palm – the receiver – and the right hand the positive palm – the transmitter. If you begin with your right hand at the base of your spine, the energy will run from bottom to top. Run it for three minutes then reverse the polarities. (It's even nicer if you can get a friend to do it for you. I always think self-healing is a bit like masturbation – practical and time-saving but not nearly as much fun as playing with someone else.) This exercise is a handy first-aid procedure if you're feeling torpid. I've used it many times since and it really works.

Here's another extremely effective one for discharging tension in the neck and shoulders: Place one hand flat on the solar plexus just below the ribcage, and the other with fingers spread out along the neck vertebrae as if you were playing the piano. (Hold for about five minutes.) I've done this on myself and on others and people invariably report a lovely feeling of warmth and ease.

And finally, as I was complaining about the uncomfortable chairs we were having to sit on, he showed me how to get rid of lower back pain. Lying on the floor with knees bent and the small of the back flat on the ground, press with rigid fingers of both hands into the two plexus points on either side of the navel.

We talked some more about finding the jewel in the molasses. How do you reach it? How do you begin to radiate outwards again? The answer is to generate heat. The treacly sludge first becomes translucent then finally transparent so that the colours of your jewel can once again shine forth.

'I use excitement to stir up the denser energies of my being so that I continually change with the world about me,' says Jack. 'In this way I never stagnate and therefore never oppose life's continuous changes. Stagnation leads to fear, doubt and anger and eventually results in disease.'

Apart from the tools of excitement and enthusiasm, the Tibetan eye-rolling is a good trick to learn. (I think I followed this bit correctly but it got rather esoteric at this point. Again, Jack's anatomical illustrations are meant to be taken figuratively rather than literally.) You turn your eyeballs up and close eyelids. Shut yourself off and focus towards the third eye. Light energy, says Jack, enters via the pineal gland where clusters of pyramid-shaped cells reflect it to the pituitary – which, in turn, functions as a prism sending the light energy down the spine through the chakras.

Most people doing this exercise feel that they're looking down a tunnel to a bright light. 'The tunnel you're looking down is your spine!' crowed Jack, richocheting round the room like a boomerang. 'You're looking at your pilot light! Your kundalini!

Your rocket engines! The light on the gonads is ready to be fired!' He was having such a thrilling time that the rest of us got carried along. 'Heat up your molasses!' he hollered.

Now we tried some 'jewel breathing' exercises. You conjure up and hold the image of a jewel in your mind's eye. Don't worry if it wants to change into a different jewel – just let it, and all the while keep up the rhythm of deep, slow alpha/theta breathing.

We discussed the properties of the various jewel colours and the clues they give you to your inner state if you can really let your imagery run wild. The mind has such a rich life of its own that sometimes I feel I only partly own mine and that it's much smarter and more artistic than I am . The jewel breathing made me very aware of this duality – part of me was creating all the colours, and another part of me was standing on the deck of a ship in the Arctic Circle watching the aurora borealis light up the sky. I was a spectator, an innocent bystander at my own show!

This is Jack's jewel guide and each jewel's associated musical notes:

RED: rubies, garnets. Associated with the musical note C. The colour of vitality; life-promoting, heating, passion.

ORANGE: fire opals, dark topaz. Note D. The colour of consciousness, mind, and mental energy (the more golden the colour, the higher the energy).

YELLOW: citrine, pale topaz. Note E. The colour of the intellect.

GREEN: emerald, green garnet. Note F. The colour of evolutionary energy, growth, love, cooling.

BLUE: sapphire, opals, aquamarine. Note G. The colour of expressive energy, volitional authority.

INDIGO: dark sapphires, alexandrite. Note A (the purest tone). This colour is made up of the three primaries and represents a synthesizing of energy of the three main qualities – vitality, intellect and expression.

PURPLE: amethyst. Note B. The colour of integral energy.

Once you can accept the idea of each chakra resonating with a particular colour, sound and frequency, you can see how colour and sound can be used therapeutically to stimulate and balance the activity of particular chakras.

Colours are also a useful tool for diagnosing your pain, both mental and physical. Jack showed us some interesting drawing exercises to illustrate this. We were each given a box of crayons and some sheets of paper. Then we were asked to pick a crayon without looking and to draw, with eyes closed, a representation of any pain we might be feeling. Jack was very good at interpreting the clues, extemporizing on the themes, and using the information they disclosed to home in on the real trouble – which might be quite different from the one you thought you were illustrating.

For example: one man unconsciously chose a brown crayon and innocently drew a jagged spiral to illustrate a nagging lower back pain.

'A perfect drawing of a spastic colon,' said Jack. 'Repressing your creativity, repressing your sexual arousal, trying to fit into preconceived models made by others' expectations. The physical constipation mirrors the emotional constipation. Are you constipated, by the way?' The poor chap, amazed, acknowledged that he had indeed been sitting on a brick for several days. 'Even the unconscious choice of brown', Jack went on relentlessly, 'shows that you have a whole lot of clearing out to do.' He prescribed some medicinal herbs to get him started.

'Pain is a marvellous alarm system,' he continued. 'It's not something to avoid, but is, in fact, a short circuit designed to let you know when something is out of harmony – something to recognize and deal with. It's a demanding discipline to be always very much aware of what your body is saying to you, to be able to listen to what your active needs are and to distinguish them from your wants.'

In addition to the unconscious drawings which revealed the hidden complexities of our beings, we each did another with eyes open and a deliberate choice of coloured crayon. These gave clues to more obvious and accessible problems.

We learned another technique calling on the power of the imagination; a variation of the jewel breathing (which is used for diagnosis). This is colour visualization breathing, used as an additional booster for self-healing. Choosing a colour helpful to your condition, visualize it as a cloud which you breathe in while slowly raising the arms in a relaxed yawning gesture. The radiantly coloured breath then travels rapidly upward just beneath the surface of the skin, rising in a spiral about the body and ending above the head in a brilliant swirl of cleansing transmuting colour. Then exhale gently, feeling the coloured breath pass out through the pores of the skin carrying all impurities with it. This is easier to do than it sounds.

I have tried it to remarkable effect with headaches and muscle tensions. The therapeutic properties of the colours according to Jack are:

RED: Good for circulation, blood ailments and paralysis.

ORANGE: Good for lactation, pulse rate, dispelling kidney stones and gallstones, hernias, appendicitis, depression.

YELLOW: Energy for the lymphatic system, good for indigestion, diabetes, kidney and liver ailments, constipation, some eye and throat infections.

GREEN: Good for nervous conditions, hay fever, ulcers, influenza, syphilis, malaria, colds.

BLUE: For pain relief, bleeding, healing burns, treating dysentery, colic, respiratory problems, skin troubles, and rheumatism.

INDIGO: Cataracts, migraine, deafness, skin disorders; has a soothing effect on eyes, ears, and nervous system.

VIOLET: Good for emotional problems, arthritis, and easing childbirth.

MAGENTA: Good for heart and mental problems.

TURQUOISE: Anti-inflammatory.

I had occasion to put this technique to the test recently. Following surgery for breast cancer, my friend Lynne was given radiation treatment to ensure the destruction of any possible remaining malignant cells. The trouble with violent drastic treatments such as chemotherapy and radiation therapy is that they destroy normal cells as well as cancer cells. The side-effects can seriously damage the body's natural ability to rally an immune response.

Lynne felt ghastly. Her poor breast looked like that of a Hiroshima survivor. I offered my services and together we reckoned that trying to mobilize her own body's defences would be the best way to help counteract the injurious effects of the radiation.

I decided to try Rosalyn Bruyere's healing wheel technique combined with getting Lynne to do colour breathing simultaneously in cooling, soothing shades of blue and turquoise.

I laid my hands on her and instantly felt an alarming unpleasant prickly sensation. All her energy seemed to be radioactive and disturbed. It was interesting to feel the turmoil so clearly. I did a general 'chelation', connecting up the joints and the chakras as Rosalyn had demonstrated, and then formed a wheel of my own energy and hers, getting the flow to circulate through both of us and discharge the harmful toxins into the earth.

It was a bit like a transfusion and a very powerful sensation for me. She, for her part, had great success with the blue breathing and immediately felt its beneficial effects.

Over the next week, she did the breathing every day on her own and then we had one more healing wheel session together. There's no rational explanation for this but we both knew instantly, and without a shadow of a doubt, that all the adverse effects were gone from her body and so was the cancer. She looked quite different and felt clean again, free of pollution, with new green shoots of life where the devastation of battle had raged.

Of course, this isn't conclusive proof of anything, but I think it illustrates how you can help the medical profession to help you by adding the power of your mind to stimulate and strengthen your recuperative processes.

The next skill on Jack's agenda was a technique he called 'Psi-phoning' – a made-up word of his from psi (things to do with the paranormal) and siphoning. It's a sort of mental run-through of any scenario that's bothering you – a preview that helps to dispel anxieties about forthcoming frightening events or uncharted waters in your life. 'Sounding out your higher self,' is how Jack puts it. 'Meditation is the mediator between you and the universe. Suck on the siphon and the universal energy tank keeps on flowing into your own personal tank. Suddenly you know what to do.'

I like this concept of making oneself receptive to the possibility of help and guidance – it's another example of surrender and trust. 'This is the exact opposite of that useless activity known as "worry",' said Jack. 'An old Celtic word meaning "strangle", causing stagnation in the throat, leading to malfunction in the thyroid (which regulates your metabolism). It also causes deficiencies in calcium and magnesium, and difficulties in communication. Your heart speeds up, your breathing becomes shallow, and just when you need oxygen in the brain, you don't get it.'

Along with all the breathing and visualizations which figure so strongly in Jack's healing philosophy is his parallel insistence on achieving and maintaining a proper balance of nutrients – cell-salts, minerals, herbs and vitamins – in the body.

'Your mind can do anything,' he said, 'but it can only achieve its goals if the body is in a physiologically balanced state and an electromagnetically balanced condition.

'When the body is not receiving sufficient nourishment it cannot achieve homeostasis,' he continued. 'It's no use just following an all-purpose diet; you have to listen to your body and tune in to its individual needs. For example, with certain types of depression, some people get sore gums, physical tics, itching on their bodies, painful joints and ringing in their ears. I can think of a hundred and fifty symptoms right off-hand where the main problem is a potassium deficiency! The patient may even crave bananas which are a good source of potassium but probably doesn't realize his body is speaking to him.'

It was a long time before medical science discovered how

dramatically certain 'killer' diseases such as scurvy and pellagra respond to a dose of vitamins, a lemon or a watercress sandwich, and most of us are still pretty ignorant of the important role minerals, trace elements and cell-salts play in the dance of life.

In Jack's book *Human Energy Systems* there is a useful list of these little life-savers and their various functions. The road to good health can start with a banana; then when the patient begins to feel a bit better he can start tackling some of the other contributory factors to his depression.

Jack is a compendium of handy health hints, a veritable encyclopaedia of believe-it-or-not facts. Here are some of them:

The reason vegetarians often look a bit lack-lustre is because they don't eat enough pigmented food. Colours are very important in food and in giving up meat, people suffer deficiencies of red. Excessive quantities of green cools down your thyroid and has a tendency to dull the organism. All the trace elements are in beetroot and vital energy is more concentrated in pigmented vegetables such as red cabbage, radishes and carrots.

I asked him about Sal's hand and he recommended massaging it with vitamin E ointment. He also said, 'Healing depends a lot on your belief system. If you know scar tissue can be replaced by flexible, living tissue, you're more than halfway there.'

I also asked him about absent healing. How does he understand the phenomenon? How does it work? 'How does an arrow reach its target?' he answered enigmatically. 'Tension, aim, impetus. You don't have to tell asphalt where to go on a bumpy road. Energy sent as pure white light will find its own level.'

He let us in on the secret of cayenne pepper, his own favourite cure-all miracle substance. 'Cayenne pepper in your food stabilizes the heart and the blood pressure, it burns away ulcers and heals tissue.' A patient of his with a nasty phlebitis ulcer was cured by a paste of cayenne, flour and water. 'Cayenne in your socks or gloves revives poor circulation and added to a massage oil makes a wonderful remedy for arthritis.'

Finally, I have since tried this herbal tea recipe of Jack's for headache and nervousness and found it very effective, especially for insomnia:

To one pint of boiling water add:
one teaspoon valerian
two teaspoons camomile
half a stick liquorice root, pounded.
Steep for ten to fifteen minutes.
Drink a cup at bedtime.

At the end of the last day Jack led us in a reverie, a form of guided daydream designed to awaken the higher consciousness.

Like the psi-phoning, it's a way to tap the reservoir of universal energy. It works as a sort of cosmic lubricating oil to flood the rusty clanking cogs squeaking round in your mind and make everything mesh more easily. The purpose is to make you aware of your emotional state without getting bogged down in its causes. (To be present and to be mindful was the Dzogchen teaching. It all fits.)

Jack's thoughts on meditation, which he tossed into the ring for us to consider, I find very interesting. Our bodies are going through a continuous process of change and transformation during our lifetimes. This metamorphosis, which is the nature of life, is also a process of dying, leaving behind, moving on. Most of us are afraid of change and afraid of dying, and that fear plays a large part in the creation and maintaining of illness. It inhibits our energy flow, restricts our spiritual growth and makes us age more quickly.

We need to take time out, says Jack, not only to eat and to rest, but also to die. 'Time out for dying,' he calls meditation. Time to leave behind old husks, empty shells, outgrown skins, and embrace the changes. This also fits in rather well with Norbu's teachings on non-attachment.

Jack is such a powerhouse. Boing! Boing! All day long, like Zebedee, the little character on springs from *The Magic Roundabout*. His is not a restful presence and I can't imagine getting much of a dialogue going with him. He's a talker rather than a listener, but good, stimulating company nonetheless, and I feel him to be a kind and sincere man.

He has transmuted, through forgiveness and love, all the suffering of the concentration camp into the driving force that fuels his mission in life. 'You always have a choice with trauma,' he said: 'to learn from it or be destroyed by it. A trauma is an experience interpreted. Not so much what happens to you but your perception of what happens to you. The whole art of life is to find joy even when negative conditions beguile us into believing it can't be found. You can choose to spend eternity crying by the Wailing Wall or to go forth healed and loving.'

He teaches that focusing on your own pain, physical or emotional, empowers the negative condition, thereby strengthening the pain. On the other hand, transferring attention to someone else's suffering miraculously reverses the polarity. Willing, loving service to another activates the higher energies, gives you a finer purpose in life, and your own troubles tend to evaporate in the process. This was the principle I saw in action at the Pyramid Healers Trust in Canterbury.

'Love is the most profitable business you can be in,' promises Jack with conviction. 'Love turns base metal to gold. Love is the magic alchemy with the power to change stagnant energy to radiant energy. Loving leads to self-healing.'

It's not that one does it for that reason, you understand, but it's definitely a rewarding by-product. Profit motive aside, I greatly enjoyed Jack's insatiable appetite for life, his endearing nuttiness, and his irresistible enthusiasm. I also think he's got it right (allowing a certain leeway for his layman's creative use of scientific explanations at times).

'Don't worry if anybody likes you or dislikes you – what do they know?' was his final piece of advice as we said goodbye. 'The recipe for an exciting life is to live spontaneously, always trusting yourself, unconcerned about winning or losing.'

Standing in the kitchen making a cup of cocoa that night at the hostel, I got talking to one of the other residents, a gentle guy called Nick who used to be a dancer until he injured his back. I ended up giving him some healing right then and there on the carpeted floor. It's certainly a lovely gift to be able to offer – a brief, loving, non-sexual contact with a stranger – a gift of sustenance and warmth that costs nothing except twenty minutes of your time.

He said it made a lot of difference to the constant, nagging pain he suffered and I was happy to reach him briefly across the gulf of loneliness, suspicion and alienation that characterizes so much of modern urban living.

Before setting off to drive south in the morning, Alice telephoned a certain Sister Thedra, a fabled wise woman of the mountains hereabouts, and asked if we could call in to visit her on our way. She lives in an isolated cottage on the slopes of Mt Shasta, an imposing, volcanic, snow-capped mountain that dominates the surrounding countryside.

She would be glad to receive us, she said. When we arrived, we were shown into her little upstairs parlour with its black cat by the fire, gently chiming mantelpiece clock, and personal knickknacks. The walls were hung with pictures of Jesus and some Hindu holy men and photographs of flying saucers. Sister Thedra, a small, frail old lady wrapped in a shawl, greeted us warmly and we sat around a little table in three rocking chairs.

Alice wanted to ask her if there was any clairvoyant guidance she could offer concerning the various possibilities and choices confronting her at the time. Should she return to New York? Should she go to New Zealand? Should she settle in London?

Sister Thedra rocked for a while, then offered her wise counsel. The gist of it was for Alice to open herself up to her inner knowing, the God within, the source, the higher consciousness. 'Listen,' she said, 'but listen as intently as a mother for her baby in the night, or a hunter for the footsteps of a deer.' Trust and surrender were the words that kept coming into her speech, reinforcing Jack's teachings and underlining all the thoughts I have been working with lately.

She told us both that guidance was all around us – and all we had to do was ask. She was pretty tired, having just taken part in a great gathering of people who come together on the mountain and combine forces for healing the earth, but she took the time to give us a lot in terms of her wisdom and kindliness. Such a humble, loving, simple person – it was a very remarkable encoun-

221

ter and left a deep impression in me, out of all proportion to her actual words. There was something magical about her. How many women like her were tortured and murdered during the witch-hunt era, I wondered?

Her mission, as she sees it, is to be a messenger. She was very badly injured in a car crash forty years ago, and 'went through death's door three times'. A voice came to her and explained she was going to be spared for a purpose – to spread the word. And from then on she has just waited for that voice to tell her what is expected of her.

Every day, usually at about 3 am, she is awakened. The voice of Sananda, 'who was once called Jesus Christ', comes to her and gives her the celestial dictation. She has formed the Association of Sananda and Sanat Kumara Inc. (ASSK) and an assistant mails out a regular newsletter to subscribers containing the latest channellings from 'The Christ Council/The Space Brothers – our Guardians'.

I learned that she spent five years in Peru preparing herself for all this. The ASSK spiritual headquarters are near Lake Titicaca and members get a lot of guidance from flying saucers and beings from other spheres. I read, in the newsletter, a telepathic communication from 'Athena in commandship Astra' and another from the 'Inter-galactic council' mostly warning us Earth-dwellers that time is running out for us if we don't mend our ways and lay down our arms.

Reading the literature is pretty barmy but meeting the woman is something completely different. I wonder if it's always the same with seers and visionaries – you have to listen to more than the words to understand what they're saying. Trying to make some sense of it without in any way wanting to detract from her convictions, I came up with this thought as an explanation:

As in the case of Tony Vernon-Vaughan, at certain moments of witnessing, maybe she is able to stand slightly outside the realm of linear time. The state of expanded consciousness may include an expanded sense of now, whereby insights from the past and the future become accessible.

Her trust and faith and willingness to be of service have

activated that direct connection with the eternal and given her these revelations (often associated with a near-death experience), which she now feels called upon to explain in words.

I guess it's in the nature of human beings to try and get everyone else to see what we have seen. We wouldn't have evolved very far if we'd kept all our eurekas to ourselves, but therein lies the trap. The words never do justice to the experience and are always vulnerable to misinterpretation. There they sit, waiting to be ridiculed or shot down in flames.

My mind is a very superior being living in a primitive brain – like a king with a speech impediment in a crofter's hovel. Every once in a while it gets a glimpse of itself in a small cracked mirror. What magnificence! What glory! 'D-d-d-d . . . G-g-g-g . . .' it stammers, trying to share the splendour. Then it's back to work scrubbing the floor.

'There are things in the psyche which I do not produce,' wrote Jung in *Memories, Dreams, Reflections*. 'They produce themselves and have their own life.' He put forward a theory that sightings of UFOs may represent a 'wave of hope in a reappearance of Christ'. A collective longing which projects itself as a thought form picked up visibly and audibly by particularly sensitive people.

Sister Thedra has no church, no altar, no dogma. 'I just come as I am,' she says, 'and do the best I can.'

Alice offered to sing for her as a gift before we left and Sister Thedra said she'd be honoured. This was Alice's own composition and it was a marvellous present: a haunting melody with beautiful words sung in a pure, sweet voice. Both Thedra and I were enchanted. I never knew Alice wrote songs.

We hugged the old lady goodbye, put a little money in her contribution box and went on our way. The whole episode had a dreamlike quality to it and I half expect that if I ever went there again, I would find that, like Brigadoon – the legendary Scottish glen – the place only exists for one day every hundred years.

We decided to head off over to the West Coast, to Mendocino, to beg a bed for the night from Alice's friend, who is a weaver.

The drive was very beautiful, winding around the shores of Clearwater Lake and through the golden tawny foothills of a Californian twilight. It's been such a bonus to get close to Alice. She is a real lightbearer and also makes me laugh.

We arrived at Mendocino after dark and I had to take the Pacific Ocean on trust. So tantalizing to hear it but not see it.

Debra, the weaver, wasn't a bit perturbed by our unannounced arrival and fixed up two mattresses on the floor. We sat around talking for a while then crashed out to the mournful sound of a buoy warning the passing ships. I'm rather glad I didn't do all this when I was younger. Middle-age gives it a wonderful extra dimension.

I peeked outside just before the sun came up and knew the day was going to be perfect. There are no curtains on Debra's windows, just a giant fir tree and the ocean. I couldn't wait to get outside and ran down on to the headland just as the sunrise hit me right between the eyes. I felt very moved and emotional. All alone by the crashing breakers of the mighty Pacific I lifted my arms. My shadow looked twenty feet tall in the long slanting rays of the rising sun and I really felt quite delirious with the elation of it all.

Alice and I ate blueberry muffins for breakfast, baked by Debra, and decided to drive the long winding coast road down to San Francisco. I'm so glad we did – it must be one of the most spectacular drives in the world. We bought ourselves a picnic lunch and ate it on the dunes of Goat Beach near Jenner with the sun warm on our backs and pelicans flying overhead.

We stopped along the way as we passed through a great redwood forest, to lean our backs against one of those kindly giants and feel the gushing primal energy roaring against our spines.

At 4 pm we reached Sausalito and Alice dropped me at my cousin's front door. (I have some very strategically placed cousins, which I acknowledge is an unfair advantage in life!) I got in a lightning tour of San Francisco, a ride on a cable car, a fish supper, a ferry across the water, a drive over the Golden Gate

Bridge and a good night's sleep in my cousin's little doll's house overlooking the Bay.

Finally to the airport and away into the night sky for a two-day flight. We crossed the international date line on the way, and the whole of October 17th disappeared into nowhere. Maybe I can ask for it back at the end of my life. I mused about the capricious nature of time; if we can't make sense of it as it exists on this little planet of ours, how are we expected to come to grips with the timelessness of eternity?

8

Searching for my Dreaming Country

At a dinner party in Melbourne one evening, a guest at the table brayed loudly that whites who claim to have an affinity with Aborigines are pretentious self-seeking show-offs. 'Stone Age chic,' he said dismissively. 'You can't possibly understand them or presume to speak up for them unless you're a hundred per cent pure blood Aborigine yourself.'

It was the culmination of a frustrating fortnight.

I was born in Australia and it has always mystified me why a Polish Jew and his Irish-Scottish wife, unable to have children for eight years, should have sailed halfway round the world in wartime to give birth to their first baby under the Southern Cross and then sailed back again to the air-raids in London.

Having spent only the first few months of my life there, I remembered nothing of my antipodean infancy, except that I've had an unaccountable feeling of well-being whenever I've chanced to be lying on my back looking up at a blue sky through eucalyptus leaves, and presume it must stir some primal pram memories.

If it's true, as a New Age astrologer friend told me, that each soul deliberately chooses its incarnation, complete with the parents it will have and the place where it will incarnate, it fits in rather well with the delightful Aboriginal version of the gooseberry bush. The story goes that little spirit children wait around in the long grass until they see a woman who they think will make a good mother, then they enter her body and begin life as a human being.

The mother I picked turned out to be a wise choice, but why Australia? I've wondered about this vaguely from time to time but never felt much interest in the country until recently when I began to experience a powerful gravitational pull to know my native soil and explore my relationship to that ancient land and its inhabitants.

Research for this book provided the perfect excuse. I would try to find out something about the oldest surviving Stone Age tradition in the world: how did the Australian Aborigines – a people intimately attuned to the Australian environment – practise their healing, and does the tradition still continue today?

For 40,000 years they have been wandering across this vast, isolated three-million-square-mile landmass in the southern hemisphere. Their lack of communication with the outside world, while they lived in an arid and inhospitable terrain, gave rise to a remarkably successful and harmonious way of life with a rich mythology and elaborate ceremonial customs. They have a beautiful concept, which they call the dreamtime, to explain the mysteries of creation. Their stories tell of giant mythical beings who rose out of the featureless plain or came across the water from the direction of the sunrise and created the landscape and the laws. The places where they walked and rested became rocks, waterholes, sacred sites to be tended in perpetuity by their descendants. And so it continued, unchanged and unchanging, world without end, until the arrival of the first European settlers only eight generations ago set in motion the forces which have all but destroyed the first Australians. The Aboriginal population today is half what it was then.

I wanted to try, before it's too late, to listen to a medicine man or sorcerer with his ear still tuned to the voices of the ancestral dreamtime beings who passed down their legacy of wisdom and knowledge to those who tread in their footsteps today.

I came to Victoria because a cousin lives there and it seemed as good a place as any to start.

It is the oddest sensation to travel through that time warp, and arrive in a place beyond one's wildest imaginings. A land with grey trees, birds that laugh, animals that bounce and furry ducks.

I asked my cousin about the Aborigines. First surprise: I learned that he, like most other white Australians, has no contact with them at all. He could show me lots of interesting books about their art and culture but he didn't actually know any and thought they lived mainly in Arnhem Land up in the north near Darwin, rather a long way from Melbourne (the distance from southern Turkey to northern Norway, in fact).

So next I went to stay with a healer friend in a suburb of Melbourne. If anyone would know, she would. Jan is a gifted psychic with a refreshing down-to-earth sense of humour, a great yearning to fulfil her purpose on earth and a corresponding belief and trust in the powers that guide her. In the manner of many contemporary spiritual healers, she works with a lot of esoteric concepts including the flow of energy in the body, past lives theory, and the use of crystals to augment healing.

While reading up on the myths and mysteries of tribal life, I was struck with how many similarities there are between Jan's method of healing and that of the traditional sorcerer in tribal society: a sense of having been 'chosen'; having to 'die' to the old life in order to be reborn to the new (Jan was in a terrible car accident that mangled her face – she healed herself with no scarring); needing to lose everything in order to be given the gift (Jan lost her home, her husband and her child); the animal or bird familiar spirit (Jan has an almost human cockatoo); the occult visions; the ability to leave one's body and travel to heaven or hell in search of a lost soul; the spirit guidance.

One way, the Aborigine way, is born out of ancient traditions and prescribed ways of doing things passed on for generations in a 'primitive', 'backward' culture (an early explorer described the Aborigines as '. . . the miserablest people in the world . . . they differ but little from brutes . . .') and another is arrived at by a process of growth and enlightenment in a modern educated Western woman. Yet both are essentially the same.

Jan is herself very interested in the link but she hasn't been in the country for very long and has been too busy to follow it up. In search of more information, I borrowed her car and went into the city. Maybe there is no hope for the continued existence of these ancient people. Everyone kept telling me that they're not making it, their ways cannot survive the 'fatal impact'; but surely there must be something they have stayed so long to pass on to us, if we can grasp it. The baton in the human relay race? It may be a unique chance to understand the flowing nature of our evolution. I was beginning to feel quite passionately that I wanted to touch that place in my inner knowing which I believe the Aborigines embody.

But everywhere I asked, nobody could tell me anything about them: 'Try the Aboriginal Handicraft Shop, the museum, the Aboriginal Study Centre.' All run by whites.

Once in the city, I went to the Aboriginal Artefacts Gallery – a dull little shop on the ninth floor of an office building and staffed by little old ladies with tight perms. They sell a few tourist boomerangs, hand-made string dilly bags at exorbitant prices and koala-printed drying-up cloths. They didn't know any Aborigines.

I walked around Melbourne, which isn't a bad city, just an undistinguished one with the usual urban vulgarities. I felt haunted by the *absence* of those first-born heirs to the soil. Their spirits watch over the antics of us brash, loud usurpers who have built car parks on their sacred sites.

I sank into a gloom.

At the museum, it seemed heavily symbolic that the Aboriginal exhibit was shoved in the corner of a poorly lit room – a few dusty, tatty artefacts badly displayed – to make room for the tinselly razzamatazz of 'One Hundred and Fifty Years of the State of Victoria'; all popcorn, corsets and stagecoaches. It gave the uncomfortable general impression that Australia only really began then. Nothing of the life, customs and astonishing miracle of the first Australians who had been surviving there for so long, intimately connected to the land and the web of life. It seemed as if everything of theirs was viewed merely with patronizing anthropological interest.

Certainly one doesn't want to be overly romantic about the nobility of their Stone Age lifestyle, but there must be lessons to learn from such a direct connection to the origins of Man on this planet; a connection and a memory as yet not totally lost by the overlays and refinements of civilization. In their dreaming may they not still have the pulse beat of the universe in their blood? What wisdoms have they brought with them from beyond the rising sun and what do they understand of the proper balance between spirit, mind and body?

Temporarily discouraged, I wandered into a bookshop, which usually cheers me up, and the first thing I saw was a copy of Ian Gawler's book *You Can Conquer Cancer*. I had already heard of him from two sources as an extraordinarily courageous man who had healed himself of cancer and was now helping others to do the same. So I bought the book and decided to try and meet him. If I was to be stuck in Melbourne at least there were other things I could find out about healing. I would take a little detour.

Ian Gawler was a decathlon athlete and a young vet with a successful practice in a country town near Melbourne who developed a virulent form of bone cancer at the age of twenty-four. It galloped through him and he even had one of his legs amputated in an attempt to halt it. But the cancer reappeared and he was given two weeks to live. Now, ten years later, he was completely free of the disease and the father of four lovely children.

He and his wife started the Melbourne Cancer Support Group which led to the formation of the Australian Cancer Patients Foundation which helps people to adopt a positive and hopeful approach to their illness. Luckily Jan had his phone number and I arranged to sit in on one of the support group meetings the following day.

Ian, with the constant optimism and companionship of his wife, explored all the available treatments both conventional and unorthodox, including a visit to the psychic surgeons in the Philippines and one to Sai Baba, a holy man in India. His book, although primarily about the overcoming of cancer, has much wider implications for healing generally. The woman who typed the manuscript for the book was so inspired by reading it that she cured herself of rheumatoid arthritis and has now been able to return to her former profession as a veterinary surgeon and perform delicate operations. It is, quite simply, the best and most inspirational book on the subject of self-help that I have seen.

The group consisted of about twenty people in various stages of combating the illness. Some looked pretty battle-scarred, having lost all their hair from chemotherapy. Some, holding a spouse's supportive hand, looked very frightened; some looked pretty bouncy and were obviously winning. Ian is a very good group leader, charming, natural and attractive, dressed in a long kaftan. You hardly notice the fact that he only has one leg, he seems such a whole man. He began by sharing encouraging success stories with the group:

One concerned a farmer with bowel cancer. 'Frankly, Lewis, I find treating patients of your sort very unrewarding,' said his doctor, giving him three months to live. He sought a second opinion. 'You've still got your mind and your spirit,' said the next doctor, 'there's a lot you can do with that.' Eleven weeks later, the man had a fifteen per cent reduction in his tumours and was well on the way to recovery. It's now four years later and he looks great.

Ian warned that often, in the early stages of healing when the body is starting to respond, the patient experiences what he calls a 'healing crisis'. 'Cold turkey' dietary measures can really provoke a strong healing reaction and since the cancers are dying from the inside out, it's not uncommon for the warfare to make itself felt on the outside; hence violent painful reactions as the toxins begin to discharge.

The accent was on mutual support and kindliness. We all stood in a circle and everyone massaged their neighbour's shoulders. This was followed by a long meditation. Meditation forms the backbone of Ian's healing theory. He believes it is the single most powerful tool to aid recovery and promote both quantity and quality of life. Essentially, it works because it stills the active, thinking brain and allows the creative, intuitive side to come into its own. Significantly, the very act of trying too hard will often result in failure. Only by abandoning our usual sense of striving and achievement – being passive and trusting for a change – do we allow ourselves to be open, really open, to the principles of change. We are so used to struggling for things that it's quite difficult to learn that meditation works best when it's effortless. All you need to do is make time for it.

Today's class – the fifth out of twelve weekly sessions covering various topics such as stress, healing techniques, relaxation and pain control – was to do with food management, good diet, tasty ways of using some of the ingredients and the whole psychological importance of taking this basic step in self-determination.

Certain foods are known to be carcinogenic or doubtfully beneficial to cancer patients so he talked about ways of experimenting to find out what suits your body, coming to terms with it, and then trying not to be too paranoid about it. People who put effort into their diets really get rewards, he said. Convince yourself you're doing the right thing, especially if you're a new patient in the first few months, and then you can allow yourself a little latitude. These were some of the tips which came out in the discussion:

Try doing without dairy products, eggs and meat to see if you feel better. Eat as many raw foods as you can. Be mindful of getting enough energy from carbohydrates. Get organically grown things if you can. Coffee and tea are best avoided. Eat tofu (a curd made from soya milk) which is bland and easily digested (sprinkled with ginger and soy sauce and cooked in the oven was one suggestion). Miso soup with seaweed, carrots, pumpkin and little blocks of tofu is 'very good if you've had chemotherapy and are feeling yuk'. Use almonds (soaked overnight to make them more digestible) and pumpkin seeds liquidized in a blender together to make a tasty almond butter very high in zinc which is good for you. Be careful of sunflower seeds as they go rancid – rancid oils are carcinogenic and interfere with the auto-immune system.

Try sprouting your own seeds, alfalfa, fenugreek, etc. Fenugreek has a lot of sulphur in it – a good blood cleanser. So is a drink made from wheat grass. Having your own flour mill was highly recommended, a great gadget which produces superb flour for bread and grinds oats for porridge. The best possible start to the day is porridge slow-cooked overnight with sun-dried currants, brewer's yeast, almonds, dolomite, and grape juice instead of milk.

Salad sandwiches for lunch made with your own home-made bread (average white sliced has gone through thirty-two chemical processes). The more alkaline the food is the better for cancer patients so eat plenty of rye, buckwheat, millet, oats, and brown rice. Concentrate on seasonal foods from your own vicinity (not pineapples in the middle of winter). Sit down, feel good about your food, give thanks and enjoy it.

After the meeting was over I spoke with Ian, a serene man with the gift of being able to illuminate for others the lessons he learned from overcoming his own cancer. Fundamental, in his opinion, is doing away with the hapless, helpless victim image. 'Victim-consciousness is probably the most negative emotion in which we can indulge,' he said. 'It allows us to feel as if we had no part in the development of the disease itself; as if it just happened and we had nothing to do with it.'

But on top of everything else, surely it's no help to the patient to be made to feel that it's their fault as well. I put forward my reservations and he replied that, of course, blame doesn't enter into it at all. Cancer has many overlapping causes, not one but a combination of many factors. 'Like the camel's back, the body must be labouring under the weight of many burdens before the one final straw breaks it – breaks through the immune system and allows the cancer to develop. Once the causes of the problem have been identified, it makes it so much easier to take appropriate action.' As he writes in his book:

'Cancer is a dynamic process. It is responsive to the influences acting on it. Remove the disease-producing causes and replace them with health-promoting influences and you turn the process around.'

Cancer's causes, he believes, generally build up over a long period. There is often a trigger factor that is the most obvious cause, such as being a heavy smoker or having a high fat diet, but only in a body already weakened by other factors will it be the last straw and precipitate the actual physical symptoms. The tendency then is to treat only the symptoms rather than the underlying collection of causes as well.

'I came to recognize and accept that I was truly responsible for my own condition,' he said, 'that it was me and I owned it. Cancer is telling you to change and the disease creates the excuse for change. It produces a new situation or insight that allows the patient the space to change their rigid patterns. It is satisfying when you can begin to see disease as an opportunity for soul growth through learning and endeavour. Hope is the key here. Once that hope is revived then the rebuilding process is under way. The sense of being a victim gives way to a feeling of being responsible and in control.'

Ian's regime of diet, meditation and positive thinking has already helped over a thousand patients to improve their situation. He doesn't hide the fact that a cure may not always be possible. Not everyone will be freed from their physical symptoms and some will need to come to terms with dying. 'Success or failure is not marked by death,' he says, 'but by poise and equanimity.' Some of the greatest successes, in his opinion, have been people who have chosen to live life to the full and to accept whatever it had to offer in return even if it was only for a short time. Any effort, he is convinced, will be rewarded.

It was very exciting and inspirational to see this work going on. Such a very short time ago this approach to cancer treatment was unheard of, now it is beginning to surface all over the place: in the work of the Simontons and Elisabeth Kübler-Ross in America and of the Bristol Cancer Help Centre in England.

All this, of course, had nothing to do with the Aborigines but it certainly bore a direct relationship to the general thread that has been running through all of my discoveries about healing – healing as the creation of a space wherein dynamic change can take place.

A good diet; herbal remedies; rest and relaxation; breathing control; the cultivation of some sort of state of spiritual receptivity such as meditation or prayer; a hopeful positive attitude. These are all things the patient can achieve for himself – all healing, in fact, has got to be self-healing. The 'healer's' role is as catalyst. And whether his style is as magician, shaman, guru, medium or counsellor, he supplies the jump leads.

It was this same evening, when Jan had invited a few people

round for dinner in the hope of my getting some kind of lead, that I got thumped with the 'Stone Age chic' put-down. I knew what he meant. Twenty years ago it was all the rage in smart society to have a black lover or to invite Tariq Ali or Michael X to your cocktail parties. I acknowledge that there is a danger of becoming naively associated with 'causes' about which you know nothing, getting carried away with false romanticism and ending up doing more harm than good. I hope I'm not guilty of that but it's a risk I have to take anyway.

Jan, seeing my disheartenment and frustration, rang a couple of possible contacts for me. Finally someone remembered a chap in Adelaide called Djangawu, a white man who says he is an Aborigine and who has given workshops in Aboriginal healing techniques. At least it was a chance so I called him. Instant rapport on the telephone! 'Why don't you come down here and stay with us?' he said. So I decided then and there to go to Adelaide on the next bus. Everything in me said 'Follow your instincts'. It was a time to test the principle of trusting that you will always be in the right place at the right time. It's stood me in good stead so far.

It was the beginning of a marvellous adventure.

Rolling along the Western Highway to Adelaide, accompanied by my dishevelled and somewhat overweight reflection in the bus window, I grinned at the more farcical aspects of this Twicken-ham Housewife's Guide to the Galaxy. The bus journey took ten hours – short by Australian standards, of course, but it gave me some feel for the sheer size and scale of the country. I dozed a bit – the scenery varied subtly from hilly to flat, from trees to plains, but largely it was endless, endless sameness. A further hour's train ride out to their suburb and I turned up pretty tired on Djangawu's doorstep.

He and Omega, his lady, welcomed me warmly and we ate a frugal vegetarian meal together. I was bursting with questions presented by the conundrum of this red-headed, thin white man with a beard and long curls who says he is an Aborigine. What, then, is an Aborigine? Do you have to be born one? Can you be adopted? Or adopt yourself? Is it a state of mind? He sat on his haunches and paused a very long time between each cryptic answer.

He spoke about 'attunement' and a feeling of 'oneness' for the land and the dreaming.

Omega added, 'If ever you ask an Aborigine questions you might have to wait a long time for the answer – days even. They are afraid of giving away their power.' There are those, she said, who have been lured into white man's settlements and missions with promises and threats only to find themselves utterly unmanned, victims of diseases for which they have no immunity, and sickened by 'white man's tucker' that doesn't suit their digestive systems.

Separated from their land with its myriad symbolism and sacred ancient meanings, they have been cut off from the source of their power – the dreaming. Fences and highways sever their great ancestral pathways and the delicate balance of their fragile interaction with the environment is ruined. No wonder they are wary of being conned and guard jealously any secrets which are still known.

The puzzle still remained: who was Djangawu and what was his story? Maybe he would tell me, maybe he wouldn't. I think what he wanted me to understand at that stage was that empathy and attunement are more important than explanations. It's not a bad thing for me to learn to absorb things a bit more through my pores, as it were, instead of getting bogged down in talk, so for the time being I was happy to take him at face value. But he certainly was a bit strange.

Omega, on the other hand, was sane and strong – not the sort of person to stick around anyone bogus. She is a trained nurse who became, early on, very disenchanted with hospitals and sought a better way to promote health and well-being. She took a massage course and that led on to the range of holistic therapies she offers now, including re-birthing (basically a breathing technique designed to simulate the experience of being born and help the patient to dissolve tensions and negative emotions stored in the body since the moment of birth trauma) and pregnancy, birth and post-natal counselling.

Djangawu has extensive knowledge of native plants, nutrition and medicinal herbs, and he leads meditation and self-awareness groups. Together they have started a little Centre for Human Awareness where they are trying to put their principles into action.

We sat around on cushions with a candle flickering, listening to mystic Japanese flute music, and I had to laugh a bit to think how my children would mock this hippydom. They tend to see me as a rather geriatric flower child and this picture would confirm their worst suspicions.

When I first spoke to Djangawu on the phone he seemed to imply that it would be no problem to introduce me to some tribal people but it was now obvious that I was going to have to bide my time, which was a bit disorientating.

I found Djangawu's secretiveness and excessive use of the cryptic statement fairly trying. I tried to pin him down to some suggestions. If he was an Aborigine, couldn't I perhaps meet some members of his own family? None left. Were there any tribal elders living nearby? Not any more. It was so difficult to hold a conversation with him.

Omega could see I was getting a bit crestfallen so she took matters into her own hands. She phoned an old friend, David, a teacher in Arnhem Land. Yes, he knew a couple of Aboriginal women health workers in the local hospital who were trying to reintroduce traditional healing into the settlements. Yes, I could stay with him if I needed to and he'd point me in the right direction. At last!

The catch, of course, was the ferocious cost of long-distance travel. Darwin was four thousand miles away. I knew I must try and go whatever the debt I amassed; I'd just have to sort it out when I got home. It would be stupid to come all this way and not follow it through.

I tried to pump Omega for some insight into Djangawu's extraordinary character. I liked her very much and really admired her stillness and centredness. But she knows practically nothing about his origins either as he maintains his air of mystery even with her. There is something almost alien about him, an impression he likes to foster. I'll never know how much of Djangawu's legend about himself is imagination but, as with Tony Vernon-Vaughan, I don't think it really matters. He is a very gentle person to have in the world, and whether he has arrived at his present state of mind by epilepsy, mental illness or intergalactic travel, where he is now is what counts.

He and I will always be connected, he said, and have interrelated obligations to one another because we are brother and sister. We have shared many lifetimes before . . . Jack Schwartz said once, when we were talking about reincarnation theory, that it may be possible to 'resonate with occurrences' out of the past – to be in tune, psychically, with someone else's life as if it were our own – but that we must be very careful not to jump to conclusions about past lives on the basis of such evidence. That seems pleasingly undogmatic to me and supplied the germ of an idea I could accept.

Maybe somewhere in the infinity of absolute time Djangawu and I issued from the same seed. Strange man that he is, it's impossible to guess his age. Sometimes he looks like a wizened little old gnome and sometimes he could be twenty-five. He says he has travelled to other planets. My guess is that something very traumatic happened to him at some time in his life and that he sort of 'died' to the old life and was reborn into this new existence with certain thought forms of a more cosmic and timeless nature accessible to him. Something about him is a mirror. His very enigmatic qualities seem to act as a reflective surface for me. He is other-worldly and not quite human, with madness and stardust in his eyes. But if I really listen to the silences between his riddles I think I can begin to understand the purpose of our coming together. He makes me slow down; question assumptions; open myself to unfamiliar concepts; make new connections. Only later did I realize what an essential staging post he was on my journey to the Aborigines. A place where I stopped, rested and changed horses, changed modes: a halfway house. Like the time when I was ill in Kenya and was forced to shift into a different time-scale. Without Djangawu, I don't think I would have been so well prepared.

We come from beyond the solar system, he and I, he says. We are 'Aborigines' because we still remember our connection to 'the source' as they do. Aborigines are, in essence, the purest form of man. They remember the creation of the world and are a direct link to the source of life. It's extraordinary to hear this 'brother' of mine try to put these thoughts into words, about intuitively knowing the things which bring you into harmony with the cosmos, as they echo my own original intuitions and reasons for wanting to come to Australia in the first place. All this, he says, is embodied in Aboriginal culture.

By and large, their philosophy of life and their concepts have been very inadequately translated into European terms. Maybe there is no way of translating this knowledge into a language-bound frame of reference. We use words and rely on them to convey meaning so much that we've almost forgotten some of the older methods of communication: telepathy, empathy, intuition.

Djangawu believes that the Aborigines have this lesson to teach modern man: that it is still possible and accessible to all human beings to achieve a state of harmony and integration with the spiritual world and the physical environment. And when you truly know yourself, where you stand in relation to the source and take full responsibility for your state of being, transformation can take place without recourse to disease.

Disease is a manifestation of being out of alignment.

He sat on his haunches, totally naked, with a faraway look in his eyes, his wild curls tangled about his head. Not very good with words, he either said nothing at all or gave elliptical answers to the questions I asked him. And yet somehow he knew. Without getting too fanciful about it I felt that we understood each other at a non-verbal level of communication and shared a common heartbeat, an echo sounding from the distant dreamtime morning of our existence on this planet.

Being born in Australia has given us both a powerful gravitational pull to the great red centre of this land and in each other we recognize kindred shades from the dreaming streams of our long journey. We have swum a long way through space and time to meet once again in Australia on our way to wherever.

Sweet gentle people, Omega and Djangawu are devoting their lives and their energies to bridging a tragic gulf. They understand what being Australian really means – why Australia is unique and not just England in a sunny place. In order to live here in harmony people must find that wholeness and oneness that the Aborigine had before the white invader came.

I bought my ticket and built in a four-day stop-over in Alice Springs on my Kangaroo Air Pass so that I could climb Ayers Rock – an obsessional fantasy – and see something of the outback. There were tearful goodbyes on the morning that Omega drove me to the station in her beat-up camper. They felt so much like family, I could hardly believe that we had only known each other for four days. Of course, there was no question in their minds that we belong together and have now been reunited to be more effective in our work. Djangawu introduced me to everyone we met as his sister 'who says she's from England, but we know better'.

I flew up to Alice Springs across a Martian landscape of iron-red desert. If you look at a map of Australia it is covered with lakes and rivers and you might well wonder why everybody keeps telling you the place is so dry. In fact the names like Lake Disappointment and Lake Hope are the clue to the devastating realization that except for five minutes a year when it rains, the lakes are salt and the riverbeds totally dry.

From the air the landscape bears an uncanny resemblance to Aboriginal art – concentric ripples in red ochre, primal patterns of land and life. I used to regard their paintings as rather primitive spots and squiggles – nothing more than abstract patterns – until it was pointed out to me that they are maps, explicit, sophisticated, stylized descriptions of identifiable locations and myths, bird's-eye views showing the great dreaming tracks of their ancestors.

By this method, the young would be instructed in the topography of the landscape as well as in the creation stories and the laws and customs of the tribe. The drawings were made in the sand with a stick or on the walls of caves – constantly renewed and refreshed – enabling a person to walk across vast tracts of empty desert where he'd never set foot before. His mental maps would tell him where the rainbow serpent had created the water-holes, what the night sky looked like, where the kangaroo women sat by their campfire.

When first taken up in an aircraft to help government surveyors plot the sacred sites in the Northern Territory, tribesmen could easily transcribe their ground drawings and point out the dream-ing sequences.

Ayers Rock – Uluru, the Aborigines call it, the world's largest single stone – was as memorable as I'd hoped, beginning with a three-hundred-mile drive to the south-west of Alice Springs through the Simpson and Gibson deserts. A surprising amount of vegetation grows here: desert oaks, mulgas, and red gum trees, spinifex grass and even some greenery at that time as it had rained about three weeks before, but it was all very dusty and dry. The Finke River which we crossed is the oldest riverbed in the world – it has never changed its course, probably because there's never any water in it. The oldest fossils have been found here (Australia is full of superlatives) and the sand goes down ninety-six feet before you hit rock, so it was costly to build the unimpressive little bridge that spans it.

My travelling companion and guide was a very knowledgeable old bushman who'd spent his whole life in the outback working as a hand on the cattle stations. Cattle stations out here are huge properties – one hundred square miles is a small one, and forty to fifty thousand square miles not unusual – almost the size of the whole of Great Britain or the state of Texas. Old Bill had a great love and respect for the canny Aborigines of the central desert area and had been rescued more than once when lost. They never got lost, he said, and lived in perfect accord with this hostile terrain.

They survived by integration rather than domination. And there seems to be a moral here for us and our lack of harmony with the environment. Our ruthless drive to control, to conquer, to subjugate, has been a rather prominent characteristic of Euro-pean civilization and may even finish us once and for all. Not only individual human beings, but the planet itself is threatened with terminal cancer, screaming out at us to change in time.

The Aborigines were once described by Mountford, a white man who lived with the desert nomads for many years, as a courteous, happy and considerate people. They had no organized warfare, no worship or pacification of a supreme being. Maintenance of the eternal life-giving forces of the land was assured and achieved by performing specific ceremonies that caused the animals and plants to increase and the rain to fall.

'Through the ages,' he wrote, 'they have evolved a code of laws so well-balanced to their mode of living, so equitable to one another, that in general they live at peace with each other and with their environment.'

Old Bill kept me entertained on the trip with stories of how the Aborigines taught him the way to live off kangaroo, lizard and witchetty grubs ('swallow them head first so they can't climb back up,' he advised me for future reference), the way they systematically fired the bush to clear the undergrowth, flush out the animals and germinate the seeds that only burst asunder in intense heat, the way they always knew where to find water.

A highly intricate system of sexual taboos used to ensure that the population was kept to a manageable size for the food resources – well thought out, simple and effective. To contrast this with the town Aborigines of today breaks your heart. Dispossessed and detribalized, they look old and broken down before their time. Syphilis is rife and twelve-year-olds get pregnant as soon as they can with no proper family structure to care for their babies. Sleeping with an Aborigine woman is insultingly referred to by white men as 'rooting a djinn'. There are many half-caste children but few mixed marriages.

We stopped along the way at a couple of outback pubs – famous and welcome refuges from the heat and the incredibly persistent flies that stick to you maddeningly like drips of jam ('the only way to keep the flies off your face is to cut a hole in the arse of your strides,' said Bill helpfully). There doesn't seem any way to do this trip except the tourist way so I resigned myself to making the most of it and settled back to listen to Bill's country-and-western tapes.

Since Uluru has been handed back to the Aborigines, all the brash disrespectful jerry-built motels that used to cluster around the base of this most sacred of sites have been abolished and all visitors have to stay at Yulara, a cleverly designed tourist village which unobtrusively melts into the desert. All pockets are catered for from the luxurious Sheraton to the modest Ayers Rock Lodge to a camp site.

Everyone goes to the sunset viewing point for the famous show as Uluru turns blood red in the glow of the dying day. This is actually quite hilarious and a marvellous example of selective viewing. Over two hundred people are ranged along the sandhill vantage point with their coaches waiting, each one getting a once-in-a-lifetime picture of the great wild wilderness, the loneliest place on earth – rock and sky and rugged desert. If they'd point their cameras the other way they would get a truer picture – a mob of amateur photographers all tripping over each other's tripods in a frenzy to get the best shot.

Human antics notwithstanding, it is an awesome sight, magnificent enough to transcend any indignities. You can't believe the sheer mighty size of the thing until you see it for yourself. The world's largest monolith – one single stone three hundred and forty-eight metres high (over one thousand feet), five and a half miles round the base, and they reckon nine-tenths of it is still underground; all we can see is the tip. The colour becomes more intense, like rare roast beef, it palpitates like the cut-out heart of the earth itself and then, suddenly, it's all over – just a huge brown rock sitting there at twilight.

Forewarned by yesterday's intense heat, the three of us who wanted to climb the rock voted to skip breakfast and get an early start. We were up by five, and Bill gave us a lift to the base. Sunrise was hitting the Olgas, twenty miles away, but the climbing track up Uluru was still in the western shadows. It's not much of a climb really – more of a very steep walk. There is a difficult scramble to separate out those with serious intent from the ones who might chicken out, then you reach a chain on which you can haul yourself up for about one-third of the way. After that comes a wider, gentler slope and it takes about an hour's uphill walking from that point to get to the summit.

Halfway up the sun thuds over the top and hits you on the head. It was still only 7 am. By midday, the heat here in the middle of this vast ocean of land is frightening in its consuming vehemence. I know I wouldn't last more than a few hours in it. I'd shrivel and blacken, sucked dry like a raisin, incinerated like a charred chop. Very humbling to realize that people have actually managed to live here for thousands of years.

At the summit it spoils the sense of rugged achievement somewhat to come upon a marker, a visitor's book and a few Swiss tourists having a triumphant yodel but it's massive enough to wander off for a bit and be alone.

Some of the more imaginative cosmic fruitcakes I've met have said that the Rock is 'a beacon that lets other intelligences know there is life on Earth – a supernatural energy source'. It's only a rock, I told myself, but nonetheless it felt special and I felt the need to celebrate being there.

I found a quiet place, took my shoes off and sat cross-legged on the ground. Here on the top a strong invisible wind blows mysteriously out of nowhere with no trees or grasses to mark its passage. The early-morning sun warmed my face. I don't know about 'a supernatural energy source' – certainly no flying saucers tried to contact me – but as I sat there I could feel vitality; quickening; a pregnant, patient, female energy humming in my body.

A tiny yellow flower grew by my side, miraculous and fragile. I closed my eyes and tried, rather self-consciously, to mark the occasion in what I felt would be an appropriate manner – with a great, rocket-powered, lift-off meditation, a magical flight, an out-of-the-body experience. But I wasn't propelled upwards no matter how hard I flapped my metaphorical wings. There was no thrust, no surge in the energy.

Instead I felt as if great loving arms were cradling me. I found myself thinking about all the marvellous women I'd encountered on this odyssey – wonderful, strong women giving their healing powers into the world. Giving a global, encircling, caring strength which has been quietly waiting to come into the ascendant after a rather long innings from the dominant masculine principle.

Women: nurturing, singing, holding, loving, dreaming. I was very moved by the pleasure of belonging. How lucky to be a woman! How lucky to be me! I savoured and enjoyed my own power, drawing it up into my body.

All in the mind? Maybe. But somehow I don't think so. I can't imagine having such a renewing and affirming relationship with the earth just anywhere. Like the eels in the Sargasso Sea, some part of me had come home, touched base. It could never have been the same in a multi-storey car park in Hounslow.

If Ayers Rock was revitalizing, Alice Springs was depressing. Baked and dusty, it's still a miracle that it's a town at all, two thousand miles from anywhere in the middle of the hottest part of the driest continent in the world.

The town is deservedly proud of its local history – the first telegraph station and other such triumphs of the pioneering spirit. But what they don't tell you in the guide books is how many derelict Aborigines are lying drunken in the streets. Rudely awakened from the dreaming, there is nothing here for them – no need for their skills. Their inherent virtues of patience and endurance are redundant in time-keeping town life. They shamble like lost woolly mammoths from another age. People feel contempt for them and laugh at them, stripped of their power and their glory. And they do look wretched, in filthy clothes with matted hair and hordes of mangy dogs and snotty children. This was my first contact with any Aborigines and it was very shocking to see them, these once-proud nomads of the desert, in such a piteous condition.

I was glad to fly away to Darwin and take a connecting flight to Nhulunbuy, a mining community in the north-east corner of Arnhem Land. My little plane made one stop at the manganese mining town of Groote Eylandt in the Gulf of Carpentaria where lots of 'real men' with workboots and tattoos stood around the airstrip looking predatory at the rare sight of a woman on her own!

9

In the Country of Dreams

Thank goodness David was there at Gove airport – another perfect stranger who has helped me and given his time. He put me up for the night and first thing in the morning I went over to the hospital to look for Aggie, one of the Aboriginal community health workers. David told me I would find her sitting with a large group of women and children who were camped among the trees nearby. The authorities don't really approve but they tolerate these bands of relatives who keep a constant vigil. They stopped talking and stared at me. Aggie, forewarned of my arrival, detached herself from the group and came forward.

After all this time in Australia, this was the first Aboriginal person I'd actually spoken to. David first met her because she was one of a group of kids deemed extra bright who were sent to a government boarding school where he taught ten years ago. Now married with two kids, she works in an office in Nhulunbuy, lives in the town and is attempting the difficult feat of straddling two cultures.

She was a little reserved to begin with but relaxed after a while as, I hope, I managed to get across my reason for coming here – not to pry, not to 'study', not to preach, but just to learn about traditional healing methods and share old wives' tales. Aggie suggested I sit down under a hibiscus bush for a while and she would call her auntie, a traditional midwife, over. A ragged old woman with broken teeth and wild hair came across with a baby draped round her neck. Gradually others drifted over until we were about fifteen sitting under the bush. The women had been out hunting that morning and brought some bush food for the old lady's daughter who is a patient at the hospital and the reason for their vigil. Turtle meat, turtle eggs, yams and mangoes. Yesterday they caught a stingray and sometimes, with luck, they harpoon a crocodile. 'We always know which are the good foods for our people to eat,' said auntie. 'Only when we eat balanda (white man's) food we get sick.'

Everyone tucked in, sitting out under the hospital bush. It was very jolly and companionable and rather tastier than the regulation semolina I remember from my own periods of hospitalization. I showed my kids' photos around and motherhood provided a wonderful starting point for getting on friendly terms. We sat under the trees all day, our words spinning a web from birth to death – from how to stimulate breast milk production and which foods a nursing mother should eat, to which songs to sing to a dying old person. As they talked the older women passed a pipe of tobacco around and the younger ones practically chain-smoked cigarettes.

When Aggie's children came out of school in the afternoon, they joined us. Her husband, Sam, a police worker, stopped by the hospital to pick us all up in their beat-up old jalopy and we drove to Yirrkala, the mission settlement.

The whole of Arnhem Land is actually an Aboriginal reserve. The first great land rights case was fought and won here and now no one is supposed to enter without a permit. I was taking a chance coming without one but I thought it would speed things up to apply in person if necessary. Most of the Aborigines in this area live in or around Yirrkala Mission where there is a church, a school, a clinic and a store established by Christian missionaries fifty years ago. They have been spared the worst excesses of the European invasion because nobody took much of an interest in north-east Arnhem Land until recently when the bauxite was discovered. But like Aborigines all over Australia, they have suffered profound upheavals in their way of life as a result of settling at the mission. Their health is affected by crowding, poor sanitation, impoverished diet, alcoholism and smoking. (I've never seen anyone smoke as much as Aboriginal women. It's almost a kind of exaggerated addiction.)

On the way I asked Sam why alcoholism was so prevalent. 'Because people feel whitefella control their lives,' he said, and added that this morning he had picked up two boys suffering from brain damage as a result of petrol sniffing. Aggie said that on the outstations where people have gone to live back on the land, you don't find those addictions. Young kids are sent out to hunt for their own food and to help build shelters for old people. Their dignity, worth, and sense of responsibility are slowly restored.

Aggie said she remembered the moment it first occurred to her that white people can sometimes be wrong. She had an argument at the hospital with a white nurse who said it was disgusting and unhygienic for the grandmother to be 'slobbering all over the baby'. The usual reaction, said Aggie, is for Aborigines to devalue their own knowing – immediately to presume they are the ones who have got it wrong. 'But I know baby needs grandmother's love. It's not always our thinking that's upside down, sometimes Europeans upside down.'

At last it seems the tide may be turning. A few people are beginning to speak up for the traditional indigenous ways in an attempt to reverse the lamentable downward spiral of Aboriginal health. There also appears to be a mass exodus from the towns back to the outstations and homelands as more and more people feel the desire to re-establish the old harmony. 'Our land and our good health go together,' said Aggie. 'Otherwise our people get sick.'

The self-governing local Aboriginal council has imposed a strict liquor ban in Yirrkala. It's a serious offence even to drive through the neighbourhood with alcohol in your car. The people asked for this restriction themselves as they appear to have such a low tolerance of alcohol's toxicity. Two beers, and their metabolism, which is so exquisitely tuned to the harshness of the environment, just breaks down.

We got all the way to Yirrkala to find that the old lady we'd come to see had gone out hunting for medicinal plants. A pity – I would have liked to have gone along if I'd known.

Aggie, upset because I looked disappointed, charged off into the bush and came back with three samples that she uses all the time: a bark which is scraped into water, boiled and used for sores and open ulcers; leaves which are used to rub on sore muscles; a type of eucalyptus leaf and bark used to make an infusion to drink for back pains. Everybody uses bush medicine, she said. Women prepare it for their families and pass on the secrets from mother to daughter. You wouldn't consult a medicine man for this kind of thing – they deal with more serious matters such as sorcery and divination.

Anyway, we would try again the next day to make contact with the old lady and there was also the possibility of Aggie's uncle, the old medicine man who had pushed off to an outstation. Nobody was quite sure where.

One constantly hears the opinion expressed by local white residents from the mining community that the 'Abos' have no concept of doing a day's work, they don't take care of material things, they make no provision for the future, they have no idea of time. There may be some truth in that, but it does seem ironic that the average Aussie miner or stockman, for example, works himself into the ground at a really hard back-breaking dirty job in order to buy himself a little air-conditioned suburban box, while his idea of the perfect holiday would be to go hunting or fishing and living rough, cooking over a campfire and sleeping under the stars without any of the frustrations or conflicts of the modern world – exactly what the nomadic Aboriginal bush life has always been!

Aggie arrived in the morning with the news that in order to visit Yirrkala I am expected to have a permit. I was afraid this might happen. No stray Europeans can come into Aboriginal territory without written permission, which can take up to four weeks if it's granted at all – not a foregone conclusion by any means. Of course it's a good rule as it keeps out unwelcome intruders and stops tourists coming to gawp but I hoped having an invitation from David would enable me to slip through the net. Aggie called the president of the Aboriginal council that decides these things and he agreed to see me so we piled into her rusty heap and bounced off down the dirt road to Yirrkala again.

About halfway there we ran out of petrol and had to sit by the roadside until someone came along who would take our jerry can into town and leave it at the petrol station, then wait another hour until someone brought it back and we could proceed. David had warned me that nothing here goes according to plan. At least I'm learning to be patient and philosophical. While we sat under a bush brushing the stinging ants away, it was another good opportunity to talk.

We were finally rescued by a mechanic with our jerry can and proceeded on our way to the council president's office. I launched myself into an impassioned declaration of sincere purpose – furthering understanding – and shortness of time among other things, and he gave me the benefit of the doubt, granting me permission to stay. He'd actually noticed me in town yesterday sitting under the trees outside the hospital.

Liyapidini Marika, the old lady we'd come to see, was there today. She is in charge of the Women's Resource Centre, a little concrete and corrugated-iron building with signs on the wall saying 'Grog is Tearing Our Families Apart' and 'Boozers are Losers'. The little place has a sewing machine, a cooker and a video. A few women and children were lying on the dirty floor watching *The Life of Jesus*.

Liyapidini is a tiny, dignified woman and everyone seems to come to her. She is besieged all day long. She has worked twenty years at her job – giving practical advice and teaching hygiene and nutrition. Two years ago she received the Order of Australia in recognition of her services.

Liyapidini is also a devout Christian and a lay preacher. She strongly believes she was called to do this work and asked me rather accusingly if I had received Christ in my heart.

I started to explain, in a long-winded way, about the kind of healing I was especially interested in and she grabbed my arm. 'You mean spiritual healing?' she said solemnly. 'I do this work also.' I twittered on that I understood the Christian willingness to be of service, that surrender and dedication, to be the very same thing I was trying to do but that I was not actually a Christian. The search for a sacred healing space; communion with the source of life; longing for oneness – to me it was very exciting to discover that all over the world people had the same basic goals and tried to make sense of the mysterious and the occult in so many varied ways according to different cultural traditions . . .

Perhaps I should have just said 'Yes'. She cooled off me a bit after that rather garbled offering but I was trying to be as honest as I could.

A very sick, thin baby was crying listlessly at his young mother's breast – poor little hands and feet covered with horrible scabies sores. Would I help to heal the baby? she asked. I think she was trying to test me out. I said I thought the baby needed medical help but that nothing could be lost by some spiritual boosting. The mother, Liyapidini, Aggie and I sat in a circle with the baby in our midst. We held hands, closed our eyes, and while Liyapidini prayed in their language, Gumatj, I gave my best energies to the endeavour. The baby was still crying (mostly out of fear of me, I think), but the mother looked happier and took the little chap off to the clinic.

Liyapidini then asked me if I would like to go with her and another of the Aboriginal church elders to a prayer meeting. I didn't know what to expect and was curious so I went gladly. I've never felt that prayers can do any harm. But it was a most bizarre and sinister event and gave me a first-hand demonstration of how some of the missionaries operate.

We gathered on the lawn of the missionary's house overlooking the beautiful tropical paradise beach and sat around in a circle. Five missionaries, the two Aboriginal ladies and myself. They prayed and sang Pentecostal, evangelical style, with talking in tongues and lots of fervent 'Thank you, Jesus. Bless you, Jesus', hands uplifted, faces ecstatic.

Then one of the missionaries started working herself up to fever pitch. 'We ask of you, blessed Jesus, to set these people FREE from the darkness. FREE from the superstitious cultural traditions that bind them. FREE from the work of the devil. FREE from the ignorance of their religious beliefs and FREE to submit themselves to YOUR domination, Lord.' Everyone was off in a sort of trance.

When the fervour had subsided a bit I had a chance to introduce myself. I said I was a learner healer writing a book about healing and curious to discover and understand the things of value in traditional Aboriginal methods. They smiled like a row of piranha fish. 'Jesus is the only healer,' they said. I replied that I certainly believed the spiritual element was an essential part of any holistic health philosophy, whatever name you chose to call it by. 'The only spirit is the Holy Spirit,' they chorused, still smiling. Not much chance of dialogue there.

Liyapidini and her friend just stood mutely by. As we walked away I said to them indignantly, 'Do you really believe that you have to reject your own culture in order to be a good Christian?' They just shrugged. 'It makes those ladies happy.'

Aggie was waiting under a tree to drive me back to town. I was really upset that two such venerable grandmothers had to sit there and be told they were benighted, backward and ignorant. She just shrugged as well. What was perfectly acceptable in Nashville seemed obscene and inappropriate here; insensitive and culturally aggressive.

Later I was again quite shocked to see how differently Aggie herself behaves when she's being bossed around in her office – patronized and told to run errands – from when she's with her family and friends: in the one role dumb and subservient, in the other confident and animated.

The pace of life crawled along. I learned the hard way that there's a fairly large gap between the theoretical plans that get made and the mind-blowing inertia and non-happenings of everyday life here.

Aggie promised to pick me up and take me hunting for crabs and oysters but she never showed up. I had turned down a fishing trip with David and some of his friends in favour of a genuine Aboriginal experience and sat at his house all day feeling cross and miserable. When the phone rang and I heard her voice, I asked what had happened. 'Argument,' she croaked in a hoarse whisper – no other explanation, no apology. She said she'd come the next day after breakfast instead, but by midday she still hadn't come.

Time was beginning to run out and no matter how hard I tried to be laid back, I was finding it hard not to get anxious. It was terribly frustrating to be so dependent, but only through her did I have any entrée into the society. I liked Aggie – she is a warm and affectionate woman – and I think she liked me but there is a considerable dichotomy, almost a schizophrenic split, between how she talks about her life; the aspirations and ideals she has for herself and her children, and the rather sordid reality of her violent domestic set-up, inadequate education, inability to think and plan in a straight line, emotional volatility. I never saw Aggie again but I heard later that her husband beat her up after an argument about another woman and she was too embarrassed to tell me. When I tried to seek her out, I know she was at home, but she wouldn't answer the door.

Feeling disappointed and useless, I walked off up the beach and stopped to talk to some of the women who camp out under the trees. They were cooking hermit crabs and making carved didgeridoos and shell necklaces to sell at the craft centre. They beckoned me over. One was the mother of the sick baby we'd done the healing for. The clinic had bandaged his raw feet but they were already filthy and covered with flies.

They have a hard life, earning just enough from selling their craft work to provide for themselves and the young children at the camp. Further up the beach is the drunkards' camp and young men from there often come and take the women's money to buy alcohol.

They talk about the old days when things were good. 'Yo! Too very much sick when people sad,' said one old lady shaking her head. Utopia was yesterday and tomorrow.

I wished I could go to an outstation and see for myself. Also, although talking to the women was interesting and valuable, I really wanted to be able to contact Aggie's uncle, the old Marrng-gitj (the Yolngu or Aboriginal word for a native healer). I kept hearing stories about him but no one had been able to tell me where he was, or maybe they just didn't want to. It was quite difficult to find anything out as the concept of objective facts doesn't really exist here. What you are allowed to know depends strictly on who you are and who is telling you.

To ensure that I didn't waste my remaining time too much, I thought the best thing I could do was to appeal directly to the council president who had granted my original permit and throw myself on his goodwill. I hitched a lift into Yirrkala and sat on the steps of his office waiting for it to open.

Suddenly, like a vision, a beautiful old man appeared, an Aborigine version of my father, with a long white beard and a wise, kindly face. He joined me on the steps and asked me what I was doing there, so I poured my heart out to him. He listened and then sat there for a while in silence smoking his pipe.

'The Marrnggitj lives on Bremmer Island,' he said finally. 'About an hour's journey from here by speedboat.' My heart quickened and then sank. Like a mirage, the nearer I got the faster my goal seemed to recede just out of reach.

Then the old man introduced himself — Wandjuk Marika, OBE, tribal elder and artist of some repute, decorated at Buckingham Palace by the Queen for services to Aboriginal culture. By a felicitous coincidence it just so happened that Bremmer Island was also his own native homeland and he was going out to visit his sisters there that very day. Everything began to come together like the interweaving voices of a fugue. He suggested we call them up on the short-wave radio to see what was happening. They said they were already expecting me and were wondering when I would make contact!

I just had time to buy some fruit and within an hour I found myself in a little outboard with nothing but the clothes I stood up in, flying with tremendous speed over the waves with a boatful of Aboriginal men I had never met before. We sped past the sacred mountain, Mt Saunders, past the rock that sticks up out of the sea to mark forever the place where an ancestor was speared in the dreamtime, and past the last point of mainland Australia. I dismissed from my mind a passing thought of the possibility of capsizing in those shark- and crocodile-infested waters surrounded by a plague of deadly box-jellyfish, and instead allowed myself to enjoy the thrill of adventure and to savour the excitement of doing exactly what I'd come all this way to do.

We arrived at Bremmer Island without incident and pulled the boat up on the shore. Right there on the beach was the family camp – a couple of awnings stretched between the trees, a little campfire and three or four women, one old man and a few children lying about on mattresses. I somehow thought an out-station would be a sizable settlement but apparently most of them are just family camps. Wandjuk's three sisters, Laklak, Dhuwarrwarr and Banygul go back and forth between the island and their beach camp on the mainland, living wherever the fancy takes them.

Laklak welcomed me and we settled under the trees to talk. The old Marrnggitj, whose name is Barrparr, was away attending a council of elders but would return later, she told me. They were reluctant to speak on his behalf, preferring for me to put my questions directly to him, but they did say that for about the last two years he had lost his magic due to the effects of alcohol and the reason they kept him over on the island now was to try and take care of him, remove him from temptation and hope that his powers would be restored to him in due course.

They boiled me up a billycan of tea and we dozed the hot, humid afternoon away. When the evening came they took me for a walk to see the sacred waterhole that miraculously seeps up from underground in the middle of this small island, providing fresh water, clean and sweet, right through the dry season. It was created by a snake, they said, the rainbow serpent, in the dreamtime and has made this the home of their fathers' fathers' fathers since the beginning of time. I dipped in my bucket and drank from their enchanted fountain of life.

Their ancestral family lands include the area of coast from Yirrkala to Nhulunbuy, Bremmer Island and Yelangbara on the Gulf of Carpentaria.

Laklak used to be a health worker herself – a job from which she'd only recently had to retire due to 'pressure' from living in the mission settlement. Everyone talks about this unnatural stress. She worked mainly in mother and baby clinics, giving first aid, teaching community hygiene and nutrition. The most common health problem in the town, not surprisingly, is diarrhoea. The standard of hygiene is appalling, with litter everywhere and scabby dogs that eat excrement. (David told me he once saw two starving dogs growling and snapping round a poor little kid's backside trying to eat the stuff as fast as it came out.) But since moving out to Bremmer Island, the children have been much healthier.

Laklak, like most of the women, makes all her own herbal medicines and only consults the doctor when all else fails. She herself had a bad back injury a few years ago and her elder sister Banygul successfully treated it with one of the steaming treatments which seem to figure quite prominently in traditional remedies.

She is also a devout Christian and combines her bush remedies with a strong belief in the power of prayer. One of the children on the island nearly died of whooping cough earlier this year and they are all convinced it was their combined effort of praying all night that saved his life. He looks pretty fit now in spite of his spectacularly runny nose and scabies sores on his feet – they treat the sores by collecting green ants, crushing and burning them, and applying the paste on to the skin. It stings, apparently, but heals effectively.

Just before sunset the boat carrying Barrparr, the old medicine man, arrived. He is a fine-looking old fellow and he came over to shake my hand. In the fading twilight we sat around in a circle in the sand and I introduced myself as an apprentice healer seeking to learn what I could from traditional Aboriginal ways.

He asked me what kind of healing I did and if I had magic powers. I said I felt I could help people by laying my hands on them and becoming a channel for spiritual power and that some things helped to make that power stronger: dream images in my mind, and sometimes crystals, colours and sounds. He nodded and lit his pipe.

His method was to use thoughts and visions, he said, to tell what was wrong, and to put his hands on the ailing part – sometimes massaging the sick person, sometimes sucking out an offending object. Perhaps he would use some special spells or one of a variety of magic stones, quartz crystals or pearl shells, that he kept in a little bag, and pretty soon the person would begin to recover. He was very interested in my large Mexican amethyst ring. I told him that some people believe that purple is the colour of healing and transformation and that the amethyst crystal helps to attract and distil that colour from the rainbow to strengthen the healing energy flowing through my hands.

He wanted to try it on so I placed it on his little finger. He closed his eyes and jammed his other fist in his armpit, then felt up and down the veins of his arm. The arm began to vibrate dramatically. Finally he pronounced that it was, indeed, a magic ring. I asked him if he would tell me how he first got his power. There was a silence in the camp and even the youngest children moved in closer to listen. Everybody loves a good story. I wrote it down word for word by the light of a torch. It went on for nearly two hours, a very involved story of meeting a spirit in a lonely place while out hunting, being very frightened, tussling back and forth in a life-and-death struggle while trying to escape and finally surrendering himself (dying to the old life?), being borne aloft and transported across the water on the spirit's back, acknowledging that he now had the spirit's power within him.

Suddenly, there was a lot of excited talking amongst the gathering in their own language and Barrparr informed me that while we were sitting there, the spirit came among us and warned him that it was unwise to speak of these things. They could all hear the spirit voice – only my ears and eyes were closed because I was a stranger. Everyone was trying to tell me politely not to ask any more questions as it might threaten his power – some things are better not revealed. Only during lengthy secret initiation ceremonies is this sacred knowledge passed on.

I promised to respect and honour his confidence and I was touched to see how tenderly the family protected him, a poor old washed-up medicine man, both from the indignities of being misrepresented by alien snoopers and from destroying himself with alcohol. We sat in the firelight, passing round the half coconut shell of kava – a potent beverage. Laklak prepared a mattress and sheet for me under the stars and one by one people drifted away to their sleeping places. There is a convention that if any lady wishes to relieve herself, she whispers the word to the other ladies and they all decamp together in a toilet party. It would be unthinkable to leave the firelight circle on your own for anything might happen in the dark: *galka* (malevolent sorcery) attacks, the appearance of evil spirits.

Privacy is not an Aboriginal concept so we walked along the beach just out of sight of the men, then all squatted down and peed companionably in a circle, chatting away the while.

People were slightly nervous for two jolly good reasons – one, that someone had been bitten in the heel by a death adder while sweeping the camp out a little while ago and, two, that a wild buffalo had been tramping about all the night before, keeping everyone awake and finally, in desperation, one of the men had chucked a spear at it, wounding it in the leg, and making it even wilder. The worry was that the wounded buffalo would rampage through the camp again tonight.

I must have slept a bit because I know I was dreaming some of the time, but I was chilly in my shorts and singlet, I kept imagining I could hear the certain sound of thundering hooves and crashing horns bearing down on my flimsy bed, and mosquitoes pestered me all night long, totally unrepelled by my insect repellent. In spite of everything, the pleasure of being here watching the silent sky revolve in splendour, smelling the delicious woodsmoke-scented air as the tide gently lapped in, made it one of the most memorable nights of my life, and I awoke at dawn to the glory of a tomato-coloured sky splashed across the Arafura Sea.

Above and around me the miracle of morning happened. Every camper knows that feeling, of course, but it seemed to be invested with a special meaning for me lying on the dawn shore of the land of my birth, listening to the whispering sounds of the Earth's morning. A thin wisp of smoke arose from the campfire, dishevelled bundles began to stir, a dog stretched, a parrot screeched, interminable insects hummed and whizzed, the tide, at its lowest ebb, was almost motionless.

In my feeling of intense happiness and completeness, a heightened clarity of vision was mine for an instant. The boundaries between temporal and external experience vanished and I escaped from my usual time-bound self.

I had come home to my earliest experience of life on this planet and felt as if I was gazing at an interior truth, hearing the murmuring of my own bloodstream, listening to that part of the collective unconscious which is stocked with the accumulation of all our evolutionary experiences. I was standing between two mirrors with my arms outstretched, touching the infinity of my soul's eternal existence – right to the vanishing point of the universe. I was in a dimension of time and space that echoed my beginning and my end – my alpha and omega – enfolded in the absolute certainty that the river of life never stops and we are connected to each other by an invisible thread. This is what Djangawu could see; part of me is rooted here with the people of the sunrise, on a coral island in the southern seas, vibrating with the myths and legends of creation. The rainbow serpent which gave it form and continues to provide it with sweet fresh water slept, coiled, beneath my feet.

Thus armed with mighty insights, I walked over to where Dhuwarrwarr was cooking a giant clam one of the women found in the night when she went to move the boat off the rocks. It provided a couple of mouthfuls each, eked out with snails and oysters. It's unthinkable not to share food – almost the worst crime you could commit. People subsist on remarkably little. A fish spear is always at the ready. Their eyesight is astonishing and they can distinguish the grey underwater shadows from all the other dancing patterns of light on the surface of the sea. But very often they have to go without.

As we sat around the campfire after breakfast, there was a general consensus that I ought to belong to an Aboriginal family and have a tribal name – partly because they can never remember 'Allegra' from one minute to the next and partly because it's almost impossible to exist outside the complex web of inter-relationships. Both they and I need to know where I stand in relation to each member of the group. A person without a family simply doesn't exist – here a casual friend is unheard of.

In view of our shared profession, they decided to make me a member of Barrparr's family; his daughter, in fact. My Aboriginal name was to be Bararrtji and Bremmer Island my homeland.

Dhuwarrwarr, Laklak and Banygul are my sisters and Wandjuk my brother. I was very pleased with this gift, which enhanced my feelings of belonging. Everyone was much happier now that they knew where I fitted in and what my status was. Even babies who used to howl when I clucked at them now stretched out their little arms.

Around noon when some of the men decided to cross over to the mainland I was offered a ride back. I would have liked to stay longer but as I was so ill-prepared it seemed a sensible idea.

In one way I think they liked me and were curious about me. On the other hand, one of the main reasons they've dispersed to the outstations in the first place is to get away from people poking into their affairs. I am an intruder, I don't understand the etiquette, and life is probably simpler and less stressful when they're not having to entertain (and feed) an outsider. I made one terrible gaffe earlier – sitting in a mixed group, I started to ask Laklak some questions to do with pregnancy and birth. Someone clapped a hand over my mouth and with a great deal of giggling and whispering explained in my ear that it is forbidden to talk about such things in front of a brother. Everyone goes to great lengths to preserve the fiction that men are not permitted to know about women's business. In reality, of course, they do. But it's very rude and ill-bred to be ignorant of these elaborate refinements.

Back in Yirrkala, I spent a lot of time sitting with Liyapidini at her little desk in the Women's Resource Centre as she coped with the sorrows, problems and muddles of the mothers and kids she works with. She is a very compassionate, serious person, and feels everything very deeply. What impresses me most about her as an effective healer is the holistic approach she instinctively takes without ever having heard that trendy word. She works on three fronts simultaneously. Using her rudimentary barefoot paramedical skills she can administer first aid and tell when an emergency needs hospitalization. Using her strong faith and genuine love and concern for her patients she attunes herself to the spiritual dimension of their needs. Using her traditional knowledge of Yolngu customs and bush medicines she can brew up some of the local remedies that everyone believes in and reinforce confidence and pride in Aboriginal culture.

She tries to encourage others to work in the outstations in the same three-fold way, and stresses the importance of going out hunting for fresh food, involving the whole family in a shared activity, and not relying on shop purchases.

She is also concerned with getting families to understand the importance of such things as post-circumcision hygiene and she counsels women not to hit themselves (an alarming ritual where women bash their foreheads violently with rocks or lumps of wood to display grief and mourning).

From having been very friendly to begin with, Liyapidini, at a certain point, became quite reserved. I noticed her watching me a lot and looking rather stony. After a while she suddenly blurted out, 'Those missionary ladies say you are a witchdoctor.' Shock! Horror! So that was it. The two fundamentalist fanatics who had been translating the New Testament into the Gumatj language had apparently been warning people to beware of me – telling them that I was an agent of darkness! I must say I was flattered that they took me so seriously, but it was a frightening indication of their ignorance and paranoia. You can see how witch-hunting caught on.

Ever since that prayer meeting I had been intent on reassuring Liyapidini that my modest aspirations are merely to exercise whatever gifts I might have and make myself into a channel for 'God's' healing power – all endorsed, thank goodness, by St Paul's Letter to the Corinthians. (I'm thankful that Bruce MacManaway had provided me with that bit of ammunition.) It was a good sign, though, that she told me about the accusation in the first place and that everyone fell about laughing. They watched me at first to see how I would take it and when I laughed they all joined in.

'Yo! Umm!' they agreed, wiping away tears of mirth. 'Nobody is perfect. We can all try our best to serve God in our own way.' Then one of the women who had laughed to hear me accused of witchcraft came forward and asked if I would heal the pressure in her head. She had been suffering from distressing memory loss and pain across the eyes. I said I would be glad to try. I laid my hands on her head and did some of the things I had learned, using colour visualization and Rosalyn Bruyere's brain-balancing technique to unblock the energy and create a flow. I felt quite a lot of tensions go out of her and I asked the other women to join in so that we were all transmitting healing energy together.

It was a lovely feeling to be linked, despite our differences, in a timeless sisterhood of 'women's business' across an eternity of shared common experience.

One morning Liyapidini took me out with her to gather some special leaves to make a bush remedy for a sick baby. I never realized how many different types of eucalyptus leaves there are in Australia – over five hundred different kinds with different uses. The one she chose was a malaleuca which had been burned in a bush fire and was putting out bunches of new growth.

An important feature in the selection of bush remedies appears to be the choice of a *particular* plant which resonates with the patient. 'Seeing with inside eyes', it's called. These were the mysteries to which Djangawu had begun to introduce me. A plant growing in a certain grouping, flowers at a certain stage of maturity, all add symbolic and metaphorical healing properties to whatever biochemical merit the substance might have. This sensitivity to and appreciation of the land and its (scarce) bounty is what binds the people still so inextricably with the myths and legends of their dreamtime and makes it impossible to separate off their healing practices from the rest of their life.

We picked several handfuls of leaves and returned to the centre. The mother arrived carrying the sick, miserable baby – Daisy, nine months old but very small for her age. We crushed the leaves by pounding them with a rock on the cement floor then stuffed them in a billycan and boiled them up into a greenish brew which was then tipped into a tub with sufficient cold water for us to be able to put the baby in. A pungent, delicious aroma of eucalyptus oil arose in the steam and we bathed the tiny girl, pressing handfuls of the leaves on to her chest and back while she breathed in the vapour. The child actually stopped crying and splashed happily for a few minutes.

Liyapidini and I both put our hands on little Daisy and transmitted healing in our own ways — if our belief systems differed, our purpose didn't. It's a definite advantage to have a frame of reference you feel comfortable with but I don't think it matters what it is. Certainly there was a powerful purity of intention there on both our parts and I'm convinced that is the main activating mechanism for change to take place.

After the healing some of the women and kids went down to beautiful Shady Beach so I tagged along. Aboriginal children are exceptionally pretty with huge, black, liquid eyes, fine soft blond down all over their dark skin and lovely hair — sometimes tumbly curls, sometimes dead straight. Occasionally, you see a child with astonishing flaxen Nordic hair which occurs quite naturally. The teenagers are still graceful and fine-featured but as they get older they seem to spread and broaden. By thirty they're pretty broken-down-looking like Aggie, and with few exceptions are unhealthy, overweight and bashed up. In their natural nomadic state they retain their characteristic thin legs and arms and lithe wiriness, but the awful town diet they eat of take-away food, alcohol and white bread gives them vitamin deficiency, skin diseases, obesity and rotten teeth. Very sad to see.

I had brought a watermelon and we shared it round, sitting on the beach. It was at times like these that I learned most about their customs, feelings, gossip and relationships.

I learned which twigs you chew for toothache, which fruit is good for clearing the stomach after eating too much shop food. They use green ants and wild honey (sugar-bag) for colds. White clay and raw oysters for stomach-ache and diarrhoea. Flying fox for asthma and TB. Goanna fat for rheumatic fever. Breast milk for sore eyes and ears. Charcoal for cleaning teeth. Stonefish gall for neutralizing the fatal stonefish sting. If a person is bitten by a scorpion or other poisonous insect, the insect is crushed and rubbed into the wound (a forerunner of homoeopathy?).

They consented to show me how to make a more elaborate bush remedy for a partially paralysed child — a little girl who had had polio, they said. After collecting the requisite ingredients from the nearby bush we dug a pit close to the water's edge, put our firewood and heaps of pandanus nuts in and lit a fire. When the nuts were like glowing charcoal we made a bed of freshwater reeds on top and poured on a bucket of water. Clouds of efficacious balsamic steam billowed out and the terrified five-year-old was laid on top and covered with sand so that just her little face was left showing.

It was a trauma to which I would have been hesitant about subjecting a child. I was also afraid she would be burnt, as quite a lot of heat could have built up inside the pit, but nobody seemed in the least worried and carried on patting and soothing her while chatting to each other. The hottest item of gossip on everyone's lips concerned the recent violent demise of a man in Gurrumurru, a neighbouring outstation. Some said it must be murder, others suicide. 'How could he shoot himself in the back?' enquired someone. 'It must be galka attack.' Barrparr should look into it, they all agreed, because he 'sees'. He could visit the dead person in a dream and find out what happened. He could see the spirit of the murderer hanging around the corpse . . . He could tell if sorcery had made the man shoot himself . . . The speculation went round and round.

In marked contrast to the everyday practical medicine provided at a family level, in the private domain, by the women, the role of the Marrnggitj, it seemed, was more in healing the threatened stability of the community as a whole – spectacle, ceremony and magic operating in the public domain. The combination of missionaries and alcohol has fatally damaged this self-healing mechanism.

After about ten minutes the women dug the child out. I felt the place where she had been lying and it was just comfortably warm. They pressed handfuls of the warm wet sand on to her withered leg and arm and gently massaged her. She was still yelling but finally stopped when they took her into the sea to wash her off.

Talking with a Western-trained Aboriginal health worker at the government clinic, I thought, would provide an interesting contrast to the folk cures, so I paid a visit. A nice girl in a clean, crisp uniform showed me round. It started out being a brisk tour of where they kept the records, medicines, radio, snake-bite serum, etc. Until I asked her, in a casual sort of way, if they managed to incorporate any indigenous beliefs and remedies into the overall system of health care they offer. 'You mean magic?' she asked, eyes narrowing. I was really thinking in a much wider context of traditional medicine, but she launched into a passionate outburst saying that what made her angry was how doctors 'just give medicine' because they think everything is caused by germs. 'They never look for the real reason,' she said; in other words, that something or someone has upset the equilibrium. I saw an interesting connection there with the Tibetan concept of the primordial cause of illness (Chapter 6).

She wanted to know what I thought should be done when people had been subjected to galka attack (malevolent sorcery). I said I thought they could obviously benefit from both kinds of treatment simultaneously – the skills of medical doctors to work on the physical illness, and the skills of a Marrnggitj, who understands the things of the spirit, working more on the underlying causes, exorcising the evil spirits and extracting troublesome foreign bodies by magical means. This, of course, is Barrparr's department, but he was once humiliatingly thrown out of a hospital ward by the matron for 'molesting' a patient when the family had called him in – all of which no doubt contributed to his descent into alcoholism.

After fifty years of missionary influence, most people here are believing Christians. They also deeply believe in magic and sorcery. I see no reason why Christianity, medical science, herbalism and magic can't co-exist reasonably harmoniously so long as each faction respects the work of the others.

In the late afternoon I went down to the mainland beach camp where Dhuwarrwarr and her kids were now hanging out. I came to ask her advice. I had brought with me from England a ring, with the intention of possibly giving it to an Aboriginal healer valued by his community. I had decided to give it to Barrparr, not because he's the greatest healer in the world, but because he symbolizes the magical healing tradition in this culture and its continued relevance in keeping people in touch with the powers of creation and renewal.

I wasn't sure if he would find the gift acceptable so I wanted her to enquire for me to make sure that I wouldn't be breaking any taboos or committing any clangers of etiquette. She nodded but I couldn't tell from her expression what she thought of the idea.

When I tried to sleep that night my brain seethed restlessly like an active volcano, trying to process and absorb all these new experiences. I found myself thinking some more about sorcery as an explanation for illness. In some respects it's no more illogical than the theory of 'bad luck' which many Westerners adopt, or the 'germ' theory of illness which is incomplete to say the least. If state of mind contributes to healing then it stands to reason that it can equally influence illness. Beliefs are merely the heritage of being brought up with certain assumptions about the nature of reality. Scientists and religious fanatics (my witch-finding adversaries!) are just as guilty of shoring themselves up in a fortress of impregnable certainties as the most unenlightened 'primitive'. Most of us think in hand-me-down patterns and accept just as much on trust as a tribal person – invisible organisms; space travel; atoms. I have no direct experience of these things – I just believe them because I've been told they are true by people I trust – where's the difference? The fact is that Aboriginal people do perish if they've been 'sung' or had the bone pointed at them. The mental anguish of collective disapproval or ostracism quickly leads to physical death if the curse isn't removed.

I went back to Dhuwarrwarr's beach camp in the morning to check out the progress of my Bremmer Island saga. The message was that Barrparr had been informed of my gift and would be pleased to accept it. I could travel over the following day.

For my second stay on the island I borrowed a sleeping bag from David and a few supplies so as to be a bit better prepared. The boat I was told first had to go and pick up a turtle speared by Wandjuk, then it would come and get me – I was to wait down at the beach camp . . . While waiting on the beach I saw the mother of the paralysed child who had received the steaming treatment. She said the little girl had started to move around a bit – the first time she'd done anything but sit since she'd had the polio. The mother didn't seem at all surprised but I was thrilled to bits!

I sat there scanning the sea for a sign of the boat, fully realizing that I might well be waiting all day – or forever, but it was a better place than most to wait . . .

It's so pleasant down there at the beach camp, a cool breeze blows continually. In contrast the Yirrkala dwellings are squalid and stifling, designed originally for the white mission staff and now all broken down and almost buried in litter, fly-screens busted, doors hanging off. Most people just sleep outside on the ground anyway, except in the wet season.

Urgency is not an Aboriginal concept, therefore getting impatient or frustrated is a totally useless waste of energy. There is no better way to attune oneself to the rhythm of life here than to listen to the spaces between events, I told myself. Waiting is such an inseparable part of life that it's essential to experience the full flavour of it. I watched a man fishing on the beach as I sat and waited. He stood motionless for about four hours, just watching the sea, then suddenly he began a long-legged slow-motion run along the shore, spear poised in his woomera.

Elegant, powerful and graceful, he tracked the fish through the waves and then flung the spear with tremendous propulsion into the water and there was a three-foot-long kingfish wriggling on the end of it. My city slicker's heart leapt in admiration.

They chopped it into three sections, stuffed it into a billycan of sea water and boiled it up right then and there to eat. Although cooking isn't always so rudimentary. I have also seen them make a sandpit and a very hot fire with rocks laid on top. When the rocks are almost red-hot they take them out, line the pit with fragrant leaves, lay the fish (or turtle) in, put the rock back and finally pack sand on top with a few holes poked in through which water is poured to steam the fish. (No wonder the poor little child was so terrified of the bush remedy. It must have looked alarmingly as if she was about to be cooked!)

267

When we finally made the crossing to Bremmer Island late in the afternoon, the wind had got up and it was very rough. The little boat crashed along over the waves, drenching me in stinging spray as I gripped the sides for dear life.

One of the boys had killed the wounded buffalo to everyone's immense relief, but another one had appeared to take its place, rather magically. In fact they can, and do, swim over from the mainland, which is very clever of them, as if they missed the island the next stop would be Papua New Guinea.

The camp had moved from the beach to an inland site for some reason. Maybe the litter got too deep or maybe it was because the population had suddenly doubled. Apparently people always come and go in this way. Even when there's no one here at all for some time, it's still a homeland or outstation. This erratic nomadic occupation of the land was exactly what enabled the invading Europeans to justify helping themselves. How could the Aborigines prove it was 'their' land? Where were the villages? Where were the farms? Where were the fences? It's just a different concept of land use.

Barrparr seemed pleased to see me. After a seemly interval, I sat down facing him in the dust, cross-legged, and solemnly presented him with the ring, saying it was a mark of my respect for his work as a healer and as a man of high regard in his community. I had heard many stories of his power and skill and, as one healer to another, I was honoured to have been made a member of his family.

I explained that the fire opal is a stone which can reflect and augment the rays of the sun in its fiery colour and if ever a healer might feel his powers were weakening, the ring could help to strengthen him again.

He was clearly pleased by the gift; his eyes shone with the light of far-off magical deeds, and although the ring didn't even fit on the little finger of one of his huge hands, he said he would wear it on a string around his neck.

He gave it to his toothless old wife for safekeeping and then everyone launched into a collection of wondrous stories of people he had healed: Wandjuk's son once had a split vein in his leg and was bleeding profusely. Barrparr had put his hands on it and the bleeding had stopped. A woman dead for two days was restored to life. Barrparr had also on many occasions removed stones and sharp objects from people suffering the effects of sorcery or galka attacks.

I don't know how many of the stories are true or to what extent they are embroidered. The significant factor for me is that he is very much loved and revered by his community, almost like a holy relic. In the never-never land, in the once-upon-a-time, he was a dragon slayer, legendary foe of demons. The reality of this poor old man who sleeps under a tree all day and whom nobody consults much any more isn't really relevant. He is a symbolic hero, and his deeds live on in the collective memory.

As twilight fell, my new sisters spread out a large tarpaulin and showed me where to put my bed roll. Instead of being off by myself as I was before, my status as a family member meant I was now in a row with the other married ladies there without their husbands. It would be unthinkable just to doss down anywhere. The taboos are very intricate. Every tree has special significance (somebody's grandfather once slept under it) and therefore only certain people camp there.

Everyone who had brought food shared it with those who didn't have any and we ate supper in little groups. The great self-sufficiency nostalgia is really rather a myth. People talk romantically about the pleasures of hunting all their own food. The reality is quite often one small fish to go round ten mouths. Proximity to the mission also means they are always within easy reach of junk food.

However, this time there were plentiful turtle eggs and I was given some to try. You bite a little hole in the leathery shell and suck out the contents – a rich and grainy-tasting yolk and a white that never sets no matter how long you cook it, so the consistency is a bit watery, but the experience wasn't as startling as I'd feared.

You can't be fussy about food and some of it is rather alarming. I managed to avoid eating snotty gubble, black lip and duggle-duggle, but I did try a mangrove worm – not as bad as it sounds – and a witchetty grub. (I remembered old Bill's advice about swallowing it head first, but that's not how you do it – you're supposed to bite the head off and suck out the insides!) I reflected that most of us are very illogical about the foods we find repulsive, and are quite happy to peel a prawn, for instance, with all its wavy legs and crunchy exterior, but would die rather than eat a beetle or a locust.

After supper, some of the men started to play the didgeridoo and clapsticks. The tiniest children got up one at a time and sang little songs in piping voices. It was enchanting. Everyone encouraged them and laughed delightedly. Every so often one of the women would leap up in the firelight and do an impromptu stamping dance, wagging her bottom with comical eroticism. Each exhibition was greeted with gales of laughter and applause.

The didgeridoo is a huge, deep-toned, long hollow tube – made from bamboo or a eucalyptus branch hollowed out by termites. A virtuoso player can get several different sounds out of it and, by maintaining skilful, circular breathing, manage to produce a continuous zum-zumming drone. It's a spine-tingling other-worldly sound that seems to enter the soles of your feet and vibrate up your body.

It must be among the earliest musical instruments known to man and sounds rather like the shofar or ram's horn that brought down the walls of Jericho.

As the full moon rose and we sat in a circle passing round the half coconut shell of kava, the teenage boys encouraged the little children to dance to the music. A tiny three-year-old boy did his sacred goanna dance – crouched over to imitate the animal's movements, he shuffled forward in a series of stiff-legged hops and skips and tricky footwork. Slowly at first, as the didgeridoo began its sombre, mournful pulse, then as the clapsticks speeded up and the rhythm got faster, the little spindly knees started going madly from side to side. Everyone clapped and cheered.

In the moonlight the children looked like little matchstick figures drawn on a rock – miniature sacred cave paintings come to life.

Once again, I had slipped through a crack in the curtains of time to some place where the fragments of my ancient consciousness

270

survive, weaving myself into the tapestry of 'everness' by this eternal thread.

In the enchanted, transfigured night-time you could forget the dirt, the rubbish, the tedium and frustrations of the everyday reality. Here under the stars, with the firelight casting shadows of dancing children on the sand, you could be half a million years away in the country of dreams.

The fire burned down to a glowing pile of embers and the kava gradually laid everyone out. It was hard to sleep on the unyielding ground with the full moon shining in my eyes as bright as daylight and one of the old women snoring like a traction engine in my ear. But I must have dozed off because the next thing I knew was the island sunrise illuminating the daytime reality of the twentieth century again. Rather a squalid sight by the dawn's early light — bundles of sleeping rags and old Coke cans, disposable nappies and plastic bags lying about.

There's nothing romantic about the reality of the outstations. They bear as much resemblance to the idyllic noble fantasy as modern-day 'travellers' campsites under inner-city flyovers do to the golden earrings and gipsy violinist image evoked by a Brahms Hungarian Rhapsody. But I loved what they stood for: a defiant pride and the desire of the Aborigines against all the odds to be once again the masters of their own destiny, connected by an unbroken line of perspective to the origins of life on Earth.

As the men got ready to leave in the boat, I realized how lucky I had been with the timing. By the next day there would be nobody there. Everyone was going to Gurrumurru for the funeral. It was the cue for me to say a final goodbye to my new family. Laklak gave me a parting gift of a delicate shell necklace to remind me forever of my hamfistedness when I had tried to make one, and I sped away from my dreaming island, watching it until it was just a shimmer on the horizon.

A friend sent me this poem, torn out of an exhibition catalogue. I wish I knew who wrote it and hope they won't mind my quoting it:

I am of the Dreamtime which is Now but not Here.

I am of this sacred place which is Here but not Now.
My people have been recalled to the Earth, Mother
of all things

To be replaced by those who do not know
That which it is the right of all to know.
Yet I remain lest one or two of the not knowing
Might seek to know.
For these I watch. And these I shall watch over.

I flew down to Sydney to spend a few days visiting the sacred sites of my nativity, immortalized in faded white ink on the black pages of my baby album. Little snapshots of that buxom young mother and that dark-haired father with their new-born, first-born, wrinkly baby, in Rushcutter's Bay Park, Wooloomooloo, McCleay Street and the Botanical Gardens. Tears slipped from my eyes as I made my pilgrimage, lost in an amniotic reverie, coming to terms once and for all with my orphanhood and the knowledge that I have to be the grown-up now. I went to a performance of the *Messiah*, which I know my parents heard on the night before I was born. They often used to sing me 'Unto Us a Child is Given'. It didn't make me sad as I had feared, but happy. A final letting go, a ceremony of thanksgiving and farewell.

10

A Conspiracy of Emotional Consent

How lovely it would have been to have left Sydney on the *Oriana*, steaming gently away from the passenger quay as I saw it on my last day. A blast or two on the fog-horn, a fine, warm, summer rain sprinkling the cove and blurring the reflections, leaving me with a dream-like impressionist painting of my native city. Instead, alas, it was a case of the usual rushed impersonality and nasal tannoy voices of airport departures draining all the magic out of travelling. I was on my way to the Philippines, with a certain amount of trepidation as I didn't know anybody there.

Chaotic arrival at Manila late at night, and thousands of people milling about inside and outside the airport building; hot tropical rain pouring; cars locked in anarchic mortal combat; honking, shouting. There are hundreds of touts, porters and hopeful small boys who whisk your luggage away and career off into the night to find a taxi – with me running along trying to keep track of my precious belongings in the throng.

Back in the Third World again – hardening my heart to all the outstretched hands. Suddenly the rules have changed. From being a weary, shoe-string traveller, I am now fat, white and rich to people who are infinitely poorer than I have ever been. I am a walking target in a land of capitalist ethics teetering on the brink of collapse and decay, where most people have only sniffed the dream of material riches dangled tantalizingly in front of their noses by rotten politicians and TV commercials, and have never tasted the fruits for themselves.

I had been offered the use of an empty apartment by the owner in London but in the dark and the rain, with an eccentric street numbering system, I thought we would never trace the address. Luckily the taxi driver was helpful and I felt reasonably safe, but that feeling of safety is pretty fragile – I was, after all, a woman alone with all my possessions in a poor city with a high crime rate.

We drove up and down the pot-holed street peering between the windscreen wipers. Most residents are barricaded behind tall gates or walls spiked with shards of broken glass, and by the time I finally found the place it was so late that the caretaker had gone home taking the key with him. The neighbours downstairs, hearing the commotion, invited me in – two young people who are partners in a late-night restaurant. They were just leaving for work and they immediately offered to put me up for the night and insisted I come with them to eat at their place. Once again, I seemed to have landed on my feet. The Penguin Café was reminiscent of Left Bank Paris as it must have been in the thirties; full of poets, artists and students. Everyone was very friendly, there was delicious food and lots of advice about healers and places to stay in Baguio. Baguio and Pangasinan, two towns up in the hills, are the places where most of the healers, and the extraordinary, controversial psychic surgeons, have congregated. It's about a six-hour bus trip from Manila.

I heard I could catch a nine-o-clock bus from the Victory Line Terminal to Baguio so the next morning I re-packed a small bag, leaving the bulk of my stuff in the empty flat upstairs (the caretaker turned up in the morning), and jumped in a taxi.

The driver dodged his way across town through the brain-blasting cacophony of early-morning oriental traffic, lurid film posters, asphyxiating diesel fumes, all eight million of Manila's population jamming the streets and a colourful array of imaginative public transport – horse-drawn hackneys, nippy motorbikes with side-cars, called tricycles, which precariously balance any number of passengers on board, and the superb jeepneys. These are true works of art – long wheelbase twelve-seater jeep/buses made of burnished steel, festooned and fluttering with coloured streamers, embroidered dashboards, lace curtains, velvet bobbles; pictures of saints, legends and mottos painted on their sides in bright colours and several silver horse mascots riveted to their bonnets. There is no such thing as a full jeepney – one more person can always be stuffed in or clamped on to the outside. Hundreds of these fly up and down the streets vying with bikes, cabs, handcarts and pedestrians as to who can cut it the finest.

Baguio, at five thousand feet, is the highest city in the Philippines. It was a bouncy, winding, hair-raising trip up into the mountains, past rice terraces and rushing river gorges. A disconcerting roadside sign declaring 'Welcome to the home of Kamikaze' was only slightly offset by the notice above the bus-driver's head reassuring passengers that 'GOD ♡ US'. We made one stop along the way at a place unpromisingly offering 'Fast Food', but in fact it was wonderful – lightning service of rice, barbecued chicken, tiny sweet bananas and orange juice all for one pound, and in fifteen minutes we were on our way again.

Arriving in Baguio – a sprawling hill town – I took a taxi to the little pension which had been recommended: a clean, quiet place with cheap spartan accommodation and friendly management but the hardest beds in the world. I dumped my bag, procured a map and set off to try and trace my first-choice healer, Rustico Villamor. I thought I'd do my own discovering instead of going around with a guide, to avoid all possibility of someone else's vested interest.

Up until this moment, everything I knew about the faith healers of the Philippines was what I'd either read in journalistic exposés roundly condemning the whole business as trickery perpetrated by clever conjurers on the naive and credulous, or in the form of testimonies of people who have experienced miraculous cures. Rather than take anybody else's word for it, I wanted to see what happens for myself. Scientific scrutiny has usually revealed some sort of illusion or sleight-of-hand but not always: in 1973 a team of nine scientists from Britain, Japan, Germany, Switzerland and the United States came here to investigate the healing claims, bringing fifty patients with them to do some controlled experiments. All kinds of interesting things happened. One of the experts, an American biochemist suffering from an inoperable brain tumour and failing eyesight, had his vision restored in only two sessions. The leader of the group, George Meek, wrote that he was satisfied of the existence of 'psychoenergetic phenomena' in daily use by the native healers, and all members of the party signed a testimony stating that in their opinion there was no fraud involved in the operations.

Perhaps what is happening cannot be judged by scientific criteria alone, and most scientists hate that; it threatens their whole school of thought. It seems to me that setting out to prove or disprove is the wrong approach. Just because you don't understand how something works doesn't mean it can't exist. I would argue that if a healer successfully cures a patient by using magic tricks, the end justifies the means. If the healing works the method is irrelevant – a placebo or a simulated operation can result in a cure because the power of autosuggestion is such a large factor in re-activating the body's self-healing process.

Western thinking is always seeking to debunk and to expose fraud, and although I agree that people, especially those in a vulnerable and desperate condition, need to be protected against hoax, I was hoping to get a glimpse of the wider implications, and it seemed important to try and understand what part the spiritual component plays here as in other manifestations of the healing phenomenon. They call themselves faith healers. Whose faith? Theirs or the patients'? Faith or gullibility?

The descriptions and photos of the 'bloody operations' that take place here are not for the squeamish. The patient lies on a table. The healer begins lightly to massage or knead the ailing part of the anatomy, then suddenly, using nothing but bare hands, dives inside the body and rummages about, while blood and gore well up. Clots and tumours are wrenched out, blood is mopped up, the healer withdraws his hands and there is not a sign to be seen. No wound, no mark, no scar, no pain, no infection, despite the fact that nothing is sterilized and no antiseptic or anaesthetic is used.

Is it really happening? I have already learned that it is possible for energy and matter to interrelate and interchange when the right spiritual ambience is operating. A Swiss parapsychologist, Schmidt-Escher, believes that the magnetic power surrounding healers' hands can be increased to such an extent that it becomes possible to penetrate body matter (which is also held together by magnetic cohesion), to separate the cellular tissues without damaging them. When the fingers are pulled out of the body the magnetic fields close again. It sounds screwy, but after all, Jack Schwartz implied that the energy of thought was powerful enough to regenerate tissue in Sal's injured hand, and Bruce MacManaway asserted that he had personally witnessed materializations.

It has been suggested that in the Far East there isn't such a clear differentiation between matter and mind as there is in the West. There is more of a gradual overlap – a merging, making it natural for thoughts to materialize. Anyway, the healers apparently have great parapsychological gifts. A patient's recovery depends upon many factors, as healers everywhere know. What the patients experience here in the Philippines strengthens their emotional and mental resolve to an extent which enables their own bodies to develop self-healing powers. The ailing recuperative system is sparked back into action – my jump-leads theory applies again. A space in which dynamic change can take place has been created.

My guess is that successful healing is due more to this profoundly powerful and as yet improperly understood fact than to any paranormal abilities on the part of the healer. If the interplay of body, mind and spirit has contributed to the cause of the disease in the first place, it must also be effective in its cure.

I had chosen Rustico Villamor because I had been told he was a very simple, unpretentious, modest man living in a humble shack. But when I finally found his little house his wife told me that he was away in Austria and Switzerland until the end of the year. It seems fame has overtaken him.

I had a list of recommended healers and I trudged all over Baguio trying to track them down. It was a very discouraging day – either they'd gone abroad in search of rich pickings or they'd died.

I came back to my little pension with a piece of papaya and a bunch of bananas that I'd bought in the market and had a weary cup of tea. I always seem to get this stiff test at the beginning of my efforts to find things out about healing in each place, as if my tenacity and ardour need to be proved before I'm allowed to move on.

I felt chilly in the mountain night air and very uncomfortable on the hard wooden bed. I woke up at 4 am and couldn't get to sleep again, just lay in the dark thinking about how to proceed. Only cold water in the shower and a blocked-up toilet. Morale at its lowest ebb.

The following morning I ate the rest of my fruit, which cheered me up a bit, jumped a jeepney into the town centre, and had a wander through the early-morning market. The produce looked very beautiful, displayed with great artistry – tiny woven baskets packed with strawberries and the pineapples peeled diagonally. I found a couple of locally written books about the faith healers and decided to follow up a few of the recommended ones.

Of the four I tried, only Eduardo Simbol was at home. He welcomed me cordially, holding both my hands, and was interested in the fact that I said I was also a healer. Unfortunately he had taken the week off as he had been rather overworked in recent months so I wasn't able to see him in action, but he was happy to talk for a while. He told me he sometimes used the bloody surgery technique himself but regarded its main function as palliative – dealing with symptoms rather than cures, and only effective in certain cases. The real healing work, he feels, is done by magnetic energy and the power channelling through the healer's hands.

He warned me to beware of the many unscrupulous, mercenary tricksters around who have climbed on the bandwagon and even employ taxi touts at the airport to prey on unsuspecting, gullible foreigners who come in search of miracles. He said he would phone me if he were to get any unexpected customers while I was in town but I thought it unlikely; the unstable political climate in the twilight of President Marcos's reign was keeping the tourist trade away.

Spirit flagging a bit, I sat in the park and read one of the little books I'd bought, *The Magicians of God* by Jaime Licauco. In it he wrote of a quiet, unassuming healer named Placido Palitayan who had, according to the author, been much maligned by vicious local press and was once accused of trying to poison their reporter.

Placido was fixing his car in the yard when I turned up at his house. He was initially a bit guarded but once I introduced myself as an apprentice healer he pumped my hand enthusiastically. He seemed nice, with a kind, simple face, not at all flashy, and invited me back the next day when he had a group of Dutch patients coming, one of whom he was treating for cancer. At last a possible lead!

All this was before midday and I was beginning to feel extremely foot-sore and a bit peckish. I returned to the market where the food vendors display their wares in bubbling cauldrons. You choose what you fancy and sit at a little roadside table – I had lovely vegetables and rice and a sort of fried latke made of grated papaya and shrimps.

Thus fortified I thought I ought to visit the tourist office to ask if they had a list of recommended healers. I knew that the Philippine Medical Association regards faith healing as mere fakery. They even tried to ban it at one time but the attempt failed when President Marcos himself was reputedly healed by a faith healer. Alas, it has become an industry and very commercialized with a lot of vultures cashing in on tourists. So what was the tourist board's policy?

They shuffled around in a drawer and brought out an out-of-date list consisting of only five names, one of whom was among the deceased healers I had already tried to visit. They don't recommend anybody but the girl at the desk suggested I go and see Jun Labo because he is 'a really nice guy and very accommodating'. Now Jun Labo is a flamboyant and glamorous healer I'd heard about in Australia. He had married an Australian woman, Chris Cole, who came here originally to be cured and fell in love with him. He conveniently obtained Australian citizenship; she learned the techniques of psychic surgery and now practises in Sydney. I tried on several occasions to see her when I was there but only ever got her answering machine. Since his divorce from Chris Cole, Jun Labo's business interests and worldly needs have been managed by his latest lady, an astute Japanese ex-patient also miraculously healed.

I also learned from the taxi driver that Labo was the Baguio campaign manager for President Marcos's re-election, not to mention international president of the Lions Club (the first Filipino to hold that office). He also owned a hotel called Nagoya Inn where he did his healing, a night club where you could buy T-shirts with his face printed on and two travel agencies – one in Australia and the other in Hong Kong. He was president and founder of the Metaphysical Temple of the Universe, with several branches worldwide, whose stated objectives are universal brotherhood and the study of spiritual principles. The front of his establishment was plastered with Marcos campaign posters and banners. A fleet of cars with Labo's image painted on them lined the drive and inside the office were many framed smiling photos of him shaking hands with famous folk. Two police bodyguards lounged around looking rather inconsistent with spiritual pretensions. A substitute healer was winding up the last of a busload of foreign patients, his secretary informed me, as Mr Labo was too busy with the elections himself. They were having no further patients for at least a week and no, they couldn't accommodate my wish to come and look. I tried to remind myself not to confuse the messenger with the message. Not all teachers, gurus and healers are immune to human frailty. Geniuses and artists are quite often likely to be difficult, egotistical, fallible human beings. If we make allowances for them, why judge healers any differently?

I arrived at Placido's early in the morning to find the group of Dutch people waiting. I had an hour to talk with them before Placido called us in. Only one, the lung-cancer sufferer, was actually having treatment. The others were his wife and three friends who had come to give him loving support and keep him company. They had heard of Placido from a friend in Holland who had been successfully cured. This poor chap had been given six months to live by his doctors and was very sick-looking, having lost all his hair from chemotherapy.

This was to be his fourth and last day of treatment from Placido. According to him he had felt really rotten when he first arrived. He'd come off the plane in a wheelchair and could hardly stand unsupported. His body weight had dropped to eight stone from its usual twelve and a half. After the first treatment, he told me, he felt very strange, 'as if light had entered my body', and better than he'd felt in himself in many months.

Placido had 'opened his body and removed clots and lumps of stuff', both on the front and back of his chest. He had also removed a large visible cyst from the back of his neck that had been there for twenty years. He showed me the place. I asked if he minded my watching and he agreed to it readily. When Placido arrived he went into his treatment room to 'concentrate' before beginning. After a few minutes his assistant called us in. It was a small, bare room containing a table, a bowl of water and a picture of Jesus. The patient was asked to lie on the table face up with his shirt off. Placido, wearing short sleeves, washed his hands in the bowl of water then began to knead the man's chest in the area of his ribcage. Watery-looking blood began to well up and Placido pulled out a couple of tiny clots with a snapping, squelching sound like rubber bands under water. His assistant speedily mopped up the dribbles with cotton wool. He did about three rummages on the front and three on the back, each time washing his hands in between. I could at all times see that he had nothing apparently concealed. He chanted a little prayer in his own Bontoc dialect with his fingertips lightly pressed together before he began and finished each 'incision' by blowing on it which, he said, instantly closed it.

I was watching very closely from not more than a couple of feet away. It never looked to me as if the skin actually parted but I can find no explanation for the appearance of the clots out of nowhere. When the chap had been cleaned up, Placido gently massaged and stroked his chest with some balm from a little tin. He seemed to be putting his best energies into this part. Finally, he told the man to lay off sugar, sweets and chocolate as they 'feed' cancer. Not to drink alcohol or coffee nor to smoke, and every morning to face the sun with outstretched arms and breathe deeply and thankfully, to open his lungs to the air and the light now that his body was completely clear of the cancer. (As with Doc Kalii in Kenya, his assertion that the disease has been conquered, his positive certainty of a successful outcome, is an important psychological factor in the healing process.)

The man's wife wept and they embraced each other. What touched me most was the look on the chap's face. His friends said they hadn't seen him smile for ages. Now he was beaming from ear to ear and said he felt like a new man. The air of confidence was very encouraging. The group left in a buoyant mood – they were going home to Amsterdam the next day. Of course, I have no way of knowing if he was permanently cured, but I believe that something new had entered his life – something like a conspiracy of emotional consent between healer and patient. A vital element of self-determination – the very fact that they boarded the plane to come here in the first place – may have activated the faith necessary to bring about that change. Many patients experience a profound emotional reaction, a spiritual maturation which sets in motion the healing process. Lessons have been learned, attitudes shifted, and the patient is free to move on.

The act of making the pilgrimage is the important ingredient. My friend Alice wrote to me once on this point, talking about the advisability of someone going outside their own culture to seek a cure: '. . . a lot of pain and disease is formed by attitudes. The body/mind has a pattern of existence and has made an adaptation to life from a stance which is often long overdue for change, transition, transformation. Going to a "healer", for some folk, already represents a break with the traditional way of being and opens new possibilities. For others, the farther afield they go, the more they are forced to leave the customary assumptions behind. There are, of course, those who feel in jeopardy and hold on all the more; however, there are others who cross their own boundaries and re-form themselves.'

An Australian woman, Pat, arrived in Placido's little waiting room. She had come over just to see him and they hugged joyfully when they caught sight of each other. Ten years ago he had healed her. She had been smashed up in a bad road accident and her pelvis jarred out of alignment, resulting in partial paralysis and constant pain day and night until she thought she would go out of her mind.

One day, never having even heard of faith healing, she saw Placido's photo in an Australian newspaper and said, 'That man can heal me.' So she astounded her family by demanding to travel to the Philippines come what may. She now has total mobility and, as she says, 'a level of pain I can manage'. Since that time she has brought her sister out here, who had suffered a thrombotic clot after the birth of her first child and been told on no account to try to have any more children and to undergo a termination if she accidentally got pregnant, as her life would be in danger. Placido removed the source of the trouble and she now is the mother of six kids. On another occasion he also healed their mother, an arthritis sufferer. Now Pat comes over from time to time because she loves the Philippines so much and finds it a spiritual tonic just being here.

I asked Placido what the source of his power was. 'Love is the greatest power in the universe,' he answered. 'It is the energy of compassion, the energy of the grace of God and faith which activate the power. You must have a big heart. Our minds are being taught little by little the wonders of the universe. Faith enables us to see beyond. Nothing is impossible in the name of faith. It alters your perception and makes miracles happen. To serve mankind you must also have humility and obedience. Not my will but Thy will be done.' He told me that an old Filipino priest once said to him: 'To be effective in healing we should bear in mind that there are only two great realities in the whole universe: the heart of God and the heart of Man – each is seeking the other.'

Placido told me that he began healing when, as a young child of eight, he broke his fingers. He had been startled while walking alone in the dark and, thinking that ghosts were after him, had started running in a panic without looking where he was going.

He fell down a ravine and fainted away when he saw the bones of his fingers sticking out at right angles. Upon regaining consciousness, he said, 'I prayed with a soul that yearned. When a child believes, faster than lightning his thoughts can penetrate to the sky.' He found that he could push the bones back in and manipulate his fingers straight away.

After this incident he mysteriously lost the power of speech, only regaining it when he'd found his true vocation some years later. He couldn't concentrate at school and spent his time lost in visionary daydreams, leaving at grade 6. Family and friends came to him spontaneously and he found he could cure them by 'magnetic healing' (laying on of hands).

Psychic surgery with all the guts and gore, in his opinion, is 'the lowest gift of healing'; the highest is 'the power of concentration and communication to the beyond. The real light shines through when I am completely in tune.'

But now he uses the bloody materializations, recognizing that their purpose is to help faith along a bit. He quotes the Bible as saying, 'Except you do not see signs and wonders you will never believe.'

'Anything you do with a pure heart and purpose is okay if it is to help a person to get well. Of course, it is tempticing (sic) to "perform" and many people are tempted, but why expose them?' he asks. 'Fakes will pay the price with their own conscience, it's not up to me to judge them.' He also feels that the bad publicity affects general confidence in all the Filipino healers and therefore many people who might otherwise have come and perhaps been successfully cured will be put off.

Placido believes that anyone can become a healer if he or she genuinely has the desire. He himself has a sparring relationship with his God and complains from time to time about being tested so often. Once, he told me, he became paralysed after an accident – unable to move anything but his eyeballs.

In defiance of what he felt was an unjust deal from the Almighty, he fought back. He learned that the mind can dictate to the body and is by far the stronger. He focused his attention on his fingertips until he could feel some sensation there and by sheer force of will and the power of bloody-minded belief, unlocked his frozen body.

As we were talking an unexpected patient arrived: a very sick-looking man from Central America. For six years he had suffered terrible pain from his prostate. He also had partial facial paralysis, making him look very lop-sided. Placido bade him sit and calm himself while he got ready. I asked if I could watch and the man consented. I would have liked to have taken photos but it didn't seem appropriate to ask.

Again, the same routine, although this time larger lumps of clotted blood were removed from the lower abdomen. Stretch, squelch, ping. Placido showed all the gunge to the patient as he plucked it out and the chap looked rather green. The whole thing only took about five minutes or so, followed by a lengthier session of gentle stroking and massage and instructions to go and lie down quietly for at least an hour in his hotel. No coffee, alcohol or carbonated drinks, and come back tomorrow for work on the face. He wouldn't take any money until then.

There were no further appointments in Placido's book for three days so I decided to take myself off to Pangasinan right away instead of waiting till the following day. From a chance conversation with an American peace corps worker staying at my *pension*, I had learned about two exceptional women that I hoped to try and see in Pangasinan. One was the famous healer, Josephine Sison, and the other a medium called Paz Navalta.

At the bus terminal, luckily, a Philippine Rabbit was just leaving so I hopped aboard for an even more hair-raising downhill trip out of the mountains, taking hairpin bends at breakneck speed. I found myself sitting next to a young Frenchman on the journey. Like travellers everywhere we got talking. He was an ex-drug addict and alcoholic, he told me, who had been totally wrecked for seven years. His life and his body had deteriorated almost to the point of no return until something sparked an interest in healing and he suddenly pulled himself out of his nose dive. Now he was here, learning from one of the healers and healing himself by wanting to heal others. He was still heartbreakingly frail-looking, with the cadaverous face and skeletal frame of someone

285

who has been very close to death; a very sweet and touching person with great spiritual openness and a courageous humble desire to find his way. 'Once you make up your mind, it's never as difficult as you fear,' he said. He was going to Quezon City, but I had been advised to get off when we had crossed the Carmen Bridge, so I asked the conductor to tell me when we got there.

I had thought Pangasinan was a town but it's a collection of tiny hamlets in a largish province. When I got off the bus I was in the middle of nowhere, at a crossroads. A young woman standing under a tree asked me what I was doing there and when I told her, she said if I waited with her we could ride together in her brother-in-law's 'tricycle'. Sure enough, in a couple of minutes he happened along, knew just where Paz Navalta lived in Rosales and also thought she had lodgings for rent, so I squashed into the side-car with my new friend. Two pesos brought me to Paz's front door and yes, she did have one room left and yes, I could stay full-board along with the six Japanese, one English and one Australian already there to learn about healing. Paz apparently is famed for helping people to develop their own spiritual gifts. I didn't know anything about this; I was just following a hunch.

I was shown to my tiny room, just big enough to contain a bed, an electric fan (thank goodness, as the temperature down there on the plain was twenty degrees hotter), and a bare light bulb hanging on a string. The little house was stuffed with beds. God knows where their own large family slept.

At supper I was introduced to the other guests. Rae, the Australian woman, appeared to be suffering a bit from spiritual overload. She had been travelling for years, seeking enlightenment and learning every variety of healing therapy under the sun, from reflexology to vision strengthening. She had been to sixty-four different countries, climbed up every sacred mountain and bathed in every holy well, she said, and still seemed pretty mixed up to me, but I liked her for her genuine concern about people and her bravery in tackling life head-on.

She loved the Philippines best of anywhere she'd been and wanted to stay and study healing for a while before going off to India to sit at Sai Baba's feet.

She and the English guy, Melvin, met in Australia when he came to consult her about his rapidly deteriorating eyesight, and she suggested they come to the Philippines together. Three weeks before he hadn't even heard of faith healing and looked rather stunned by the whole experience. He's not a terribly adventurous person and didn't like the local food.

The Japanese party consisted of members of a spiritual development centre near Tokyo and their leader, the Reverend Bahkti, who used to be a businessman until a personal crisis some years ago forced him to rethink the direction in which his life was going. Every two months they bring a party of their countrymen over for a week of healing and then stay on for a couple of days to replenish their own spiritual stock. Only one spoke English, a gentle, pretty, bashful girl called Yumi who acted as interpreter for the rest. She also came into healing work from her own personal crisis point, when a disease of the throat caused her to give up a promising operatic singing career.

Paz Navalta is a member of the local chapter of the Union Espiritista Cristiana de Filipinas, an organization which for over fifty years has represented most of the country's healers. The Christianity here seems to be a composite conglomerate of all the positive forces that can be marshalled. Anything that can be useful is pressed into service and integrated – karma, chakras, reincarnation, voodoo trance states, spiritual ecstasy. After supper we all assembled in the little family chapel under the embroidered satin banners, Paz at the front with a large sort of ouija board on a rostrum. We began with a few Bible readings in Tagalog, Japanese and English, then we sang a simple hymn invoking the spirit to grace us with its presence. During the singing Paz goes into a trance. She becomes 'the instrument' and refers to herself as such throughout the session. One by one she tells people what their message from the spirit is. Rev. Bahkti was told that his devoted studies had now brought him to the stage where he, too, would be granted mediumistic powers. He was called forward, whereupon he also tranced rather theatrically – eyeballs rolling and the ouija board swinging about. He spoke in Japanese which Yumi translated. His mediumistic message

was that we must all try to harmonize ourselves with the gre
harmony of God and that suffering and illness are in dire
proportion to the degree to which you are out of balance with th
harmony (an interesting direct correlation with the Aborigin
philosophy of life). Everything starts, he said, every trut
and perception begins with the act of repentance – not th
abject, hair-shirt self-flagellation that word has come to b
associated with, but in its original sense of serious rethinking
reconsidering one's purpose. You will automatically rene
yourself and be newly created as you come to that reali:
ation, he said. True healing only comes from that fundamenta
understanding.

Rae was called next. She got the shakes and her body tremble
from head to foot. She opened her mouth to speak but nothin
came out. Paz said she should prepare herself more next time s
as to be in tune with the vibrations. 'Instead of asking for gift:
ask the giver of gifts.' She added, "Instead of asking for life as
the giver of life and the things and the life will be given to you
flowing through you. You can be the connecting pipe from th
fountain of life to the sick person that needs health and life.' Ra
swooned with devotion.

Quiet little self-effacing Yumi was the next to come forwarc
Her face immediately filled with emotion, she stretched out he
arms and tears rolled down her cheeks. The 'spirit' told her sh
also had mediumistic talents and would be able to use her voic
again. Suddenly, without warning, Yumi burst into song with a
really powerful soprano voice that would have shattered th
windowpanes had there been any. The room filled with thi
amazing sound like a Wagnerian Valkyrie singing. There was
slightly comic aspect to it as all the neighbourhood dogs begai
to howl, but the effect was electric because it was genuine ane
heartfelt.

The two clairvoyants in the room, Rev. Bahkti and Paz's eldes
sister, Esther, were asked if they had seen anything unusual. They
both said they saw Yumi surrounded by a crowd of angels – one
holding a single rose in her hand. The fascinating thing abou
their visions was that throughout the evening they always co

288

incided, yet neither understood the other's language and each had to be translated by a different interpreter.

Paz asked if anyone had felt anything 'while the spirit was singing through Yumi'. I nodded because I had indeed been moved and impressed by the sheer power and volume of it. So I was asked to come up and sit in the hot seat to see if I would be given gifts. She asked me what my true purpose was in coming here to this house. I answered that I hoped to learn how to become a better healer and to communicate my experiences through writing. She said I should remove all my jewellery, place my hands, palms up, on the table and open myself fully to God.

I closed my eyes and tried to be as receptive as possible. What happened next was astonishing. My hands became hot and tingly with violent pins and needles – quite uncomfortable in fact – and I could not keep my fingers still; they twitched like the fronds on a sea anemone. I felt my heartbeat increase and a warm emanation begin to pulse rhythmically from the regions of both my heart and brow chakras.

I'd hoped, of course, that I would feel something unusual, but this surpassed all my expectations. Even if it was due entirely to autosuggestion it was remarkable for its strength. The physical feelings can be intense, and can bring about physiological changes in the body, when to all intents and purposes nothing is actually happening. Whatever else, that must lend weight to the theory that there are mental and emotional components in both the cause and the cure of disease.

More interesting still was the reaction from the two clairvoyants. They gasped dramatically and both began speaking at once. Rev. Bahkti saw waves of light streaming from my fingers, heart and forehead, becoming more like shafts and growing brighter. Esther described an incandescent glow surrounding me and sparkling light dancing in my hands.

Naturally, I felt very happy to be given this lovely symbolic affirmation of myself as I would ideally like to be. I said I hoped I would become worthy of it, never forgettng that whatever it is comes through me but is not really of me.

So, what was going on here? I still consider myself to be a

level-headed, sensible, ordinary woman, but there does seem room in life for one to include the magical and the mysterious without necessarily demanding rational explanations. I am learning to live with that paradox – one of Rosalyn's most important tips: 'A healer must be able to deal with ambiguity.' The problem comes when I've tried to describe these sorts of happenings to other level-headed, sensible people such as Richard, my husband. I can see 'that look' come over them: a patronizing, indulgent expression which instantly consigns my experience to the pigeonhole marked 'religion'. He says, kindly, 'Hon, that sounds nutty.'

All I can say is I'm absolutely certain that I am no nuttier than I've ever been. Nothing's changed, only the boundaries have disappeared.

To everyone, sitting there in the bare little chapel, was given helpful advice, cleverly sounding the depths of each individual's need and reinforcing the template of each vision.

A young Japanese man still very preoccupied with his own health was told he was not yet ready to be given gifts but was given instead a mantra to help himself: a word to repeat until he felt the power flood into his body to give him strength.

Melvin, the English boy with poor eyesight, was read a passage from the Bible, then Paz gave him healing for his eyes, making scooping-away motions and then bombarding them with energy. 'Don't be so easily discouraged,' she said to him. 'God loves you. He wants you to have not only good sight but clairvoyant vision.'

To end the session everyone stepped forward to receive a spiritual 'injection' from Paz, who made the gesture of squeezing an invisble syringe into the astral body. Interestingly, many people apparently display puncture wounds complete with drops of blood after this procedure, in spite of the fact that 'it's all in the mind'. When it was my turn, instead of an injection, she took both my hands in one of hers, and with the other reached up to her embroidered banner of light – a flaming torch – and sprinkled it into my palms – a graceful and eloquent symbolism. She said I would receive God's gifts of writing and of healing. Then she looked long and hard at me and said, 'You are worried about your younger son, aren't you?' I had at no stage mentioned anything to anyone about my family, not even that I had one, but I was indeed worried about him. 'He has found growing up a difficult and painful process,' said Paz, 'and you are wondering how you can help him to find his way.' I must have looked as if I had seen a ghost. 'Don't worry,' she went on. 'He is already helped; you will observe a change when you return home. Tomorrow I will give you a mantra for healing him.' She then asked everyone to join in an absent healing for him. I was quite shaken by this unassuming display of clairvoyant brilliance and by how accurately she had picked up my only serious heart-ache.

I finally fell into bed at about eleven that night and slept like a dead person after what must have been one of the strangest and most event-filled days in my life.

I was awakened before dawn by noisy neighbours going to market and a chorus of barking dogs and networked roosters that reverberated from my earhole to the distant horizon. Impossible to sleep again. The house walls are flimsy and cheek by jowl with the people next door; all domestic and personal sound effects are clearly audible. At seven, Paz came in and sat on my bed to give me my mantra. She had risen in the middle of the night and meditated alone until it came through to her.

It was to be a secret, private, non-transferable recipe for me alone to use. She wrote it down in my notebook: three little verses in a special language straight from the spirit – it sounds rather like Esperanto. I should use it, she said, silently to bless orange juice before giving it to my son to drink. It would remove the effects of any drugs from his body and help him on his way. As he suffered from possession by bad spirits, she said, this would also discharge the low forces in him and give him the strength to resist them in future.

She was so sweet and motherly, putting her arms around my shoulders, arming me with her invincible formula for exorcism. How did she know – a simple, unsophisticated country woman – of my preoccupation with my twenty-two-year-old son, who smoked too much dope, thousands of miles away in London? The accuracy of her intuition and the elegant ceremonial symbolism of her remedy impressed me very much. I resolved to try it when I got home.

We spent a quiet meditative day visiting the magic holy well of La Fraternidad – one of the first churches of the Union Espiritista Cristiana to be built ('guidance' from the spirit world in the form of a vision came to one of the founders over a hundred years ago, who caused the well to be dug). In this part of the country you can still find the old-style traditional Filipino houses of carved wood posts, paper lattice windows, woven rush ceilings and steeply pitched thatched roofs. It is such a beautiful and appropriate style of architecture for this part of the world: cool to live in, pleasing to the eye and to the heart, blending harmoniously with the landscape. The landscape itself is a joy to be in, with well-tended rice paddies, green jungly hills in the background, muddy rivers full of tender children's bodies splashing and swimming, an old man in a conical straw hat riding on a buffalo, horse-drawn carts loaded with baskets and cane furniture making their lumbering four-day trundle to Manila, women winnowing and tossing their trays of rice in the sunlight. In this deceptive rural idyll, we were advised definitely not to wander about the lonely roads and fields in the late afternoon as there had been much NPA (National People's Army) activity and no one was immune from kidnapping.

Rae and Melvin had been bickering all day about who was projecting negativity and who kept whom awake last night – not very spiritual! We were supposed to be praying for cleansing and purification!

When you look into the waters of the well at La Fraternidad you are meant to know what your clairvoyant gifts are. I don't think I have any. I feel a lot but I don't see much – sometimes an intimation of coloured auras or swarming particles of energy – nothing very specific. I tried hard but all I saw was Rae's face looming over the edge as she nearly fell in head first in her anxiety to get the most out of the experience. Apparently people have heard music coming out of the well, or voices, or seen the water bubble right up like a boiling cauldron. Nothing dramatic happened today but the mineral-rich water felt good for the skin.

I thought I had better try to locate Josephine Sison, the other well-known woman healer in the region, and find out if I could see her the following day. Rae and Melvin tagged along. I don't mind them in small doses but I would rather not be identified with either of them! We shared a tricycle ride to Josephine's centre, La Espiritista, and learned that she would be healing at home in Barangobong the next morning at 9 am. I was very lucky to have chosen that week to be there. Josephine had been suffering from exhaustion, and had announced that she would just do four days' healing after which she was taking a year off.

We walked back to Paz's house, causing some hilarity among the locals. If I felt conspicuous before, I felt positively floodlit now and uncharitably would have loved to have been able to disassociate myself from my companions. Melvin insisted on wearing his remedial glasses, punky black opaque goggles with little perforations in, and large Rae was wearing a borrowed dress of Paz's – too small – while her own was drying on the washing line. Hair awry in a falling-down bun, carrying a massive bouquet of bougainvillaea she had picked along the way, she was waving flowers at everyone we passed. She really was rather trying, always attempting to impress you with her transcendental one-upmanship and hungrily pumping everyone for the name of any new guru to go and orbit around, terrified of missing anything she might add to her spiritual merit chart. She's a kind person and sincere, just got up my nose a bit – a real consciousness junkie and a dreadful warning!

Talking to the Japanese group through Yumi I learned something of their teachings. They believe that Buddha and Jesus were both great masters in the service of God and that God is within us – 'the light that is in your heart, closer even than your hands and feet'.

'Please understand', said Rev. Bahkti, 'the folly of attaching yourself too much to outside phenomena. A change in your own heart will bring about the miracles you seek. First the reform, then the miracle.' (Alice's very words when she spoke about those who 're-form' themselves and cross their own boundaries.) Their teaching, like the Tibetans', is based on the principle of mindfulness; constantly monitoring the subtle changes in your emotional response to the things around you, acknowledging rather than attempting to control or suppress. This has an important application in the management of pain – to recognize it and enter into it, registering the changes, is a way of taking charge. (The only time I was taught that was for riding the waves and breathing with the contractions of childbirth, but I have since found it helpful with all kinds of other pain – stomach cramps, migraine and toothache.) It is a natural law, says Yumi, that pain will begin to diminish of its own accord if you go with it. We are too afraid of the forces in our own bodies and always try to dominate them with our wills, whereas an acceptance and ownership of those forces is the only way to live fully in harmony. Ian Gawler, the cancer self-help teacher in Melbourne, said in his book *You Can Conquer Cancer*, 'Of my inner resources, I feel the most significant was an ability to see the disease as a process. As soon as it appeared, I felt that it was a product of my past actions. Recognizing that I had been involved in causing it, I felt confident that I could play a major role in getting over it. I accepted responsibility for my condition and therefore I felt in control of it.' He also says in the chapter on pain control, 'If you can accept and flow with the pain rather than resisting and struggling against it, it will cause little inconvenience.'

Yumi continued, 'It is not outside events but our perception of them that really affects us – this is what Rev. Bahkti means about not attaching yourself too much to outside phenomena – it is the changes in your own heart that govern the way life treats you. Direct your mind inward, be aware of the way in which you are responding and you will see that the answers to your questions and the solution to your problems lie within you.' ('Half the understanding of the answer is in the question,' said Tony Vernon-Vaughan. There is certainly a continuous thread in these ideas – they appear in different disguises all over the place.)

Rae had the nerve to butt in and tell Rev. Bahkti helpfully in her loud, blunt Australian tones that if he was interested she could introduce him to a 'psychic surgeon' who would teach him 'the tricks of the trade'. He declined gracefully.

I should have kept my mouth shut about visiting Josephine. The consequence of not doing so was, of course, my having to go with Rae and Melvin, my embarrassing associates. Everybody thought we were three friends travelling together!

We arrived at Barangobong by jeepney in time for the scheduled 9 am start at the little chapel attached to Josephine's house, but she didn't actually turn up until ten-thirty. In the meantime, as each person seeking treatment arrived, their name was put on a list. I was immediately cornered by Josephine's assistant, a rather pushy chap who gave me a run-down of his credentials and told me how his speciality was protecting people from the effects of black magic. He was also trying to flog his special preparation of sixty efficacious herbs in coconut oil. He told me he was also able to perform psychic surgery but I didn't see him do any. All he did was mop up blood.

Josephine herself is an amiable, pleasant woman of my age. I soon saw why she would need a rest. During the time we were waiting, the place began to fill up. More and more people packed the tiny chapel – mostly poor Filipinos, but also an Indian woman from Bihar suffering from asthma, who had never before left India but had heard of Josephine from a satisfied ex-patient and had been brought here by her husband, and two young Indian men from Calcutta bringing their brother – a poor wasted-looking fellow suffering from muscular dystrophy whom they carried in on a stretcher. All were in a state of great excitement and expectancy.

I introduced myself to Josephine and asked if I could watch and take photographs. She agreed, so long as I didn't 'disturb the vibrations'. Rae and Melvin put themselves on the list of patients.

Everyone sat on wooden benches in the chapel at the front of which was a raised portion with a green plastic-covered operating table on it, and a vase of dusty wax flowers. Behind Josephine's head was a sign stating 'God does the work, I am only His instrument; please pray.' Another gave directives to be adhered to after receiving healing: 'Do not eat meat or anything sour or cold. Do not smoke or drink alcohol. Do not take a bath or shower (sponge with luke-warm water). Rest. Do not exert strenuous effort. Refrain from romance (!). Eat vegetables, salad and fresh fruit. Drink fruit juice. Pray and Relax. Be at Peace.' I was especially interested in one notice which said people would not get better unless they changed their ways. 'The old lifestyle created the problem in the first place and it will only go away if you ask forgiveness and begin afresh. Instantaneous cures are very rare but not impossible.'

All the operations are performed with lightning speed in full view of everyone, except in a few cases where the nature of the complaint is very personal; then a cursory curtain is whipped across, but there are still people wandering about, so privacy is a bit of a lost cause.

From my seat in the front row I still couldn't really see closely enough so I asked if I could stand beside the table. Josephine, wearing a short-sleeved dress, with only a large bucket of water for washing her hands and a waste bin for chucking the gore into, began her operations. She gave most cases a quick rummage and pulled out clots, like Placido, but every once in a while she would pull out great wads of what looked like leaf compost or coconut matting and, on one occasion, a length of bloody cloth.

There would be a great gasp from all the onlookers and, as the offending material was flung away, Josephine would triumphantly say 'Black magic'. It was great theatre. She pulled a disgusting worm out of someone's eye, stones from someone's kidneys and enormous lumps of clotted gunge from the throat of a woman who had completely lost her voice for over two years. I heard that patient cry out with astonishment as she realized she could speak again.

Another extraordinary sight is her famous cotton-wool routine. She breaks off small wads from a normal commercial roll, soaks them in consecrated coconut oil and appears to dematerialize them right through the skin. Sometimes, as in the case of a little girl with a chest complaint, she leaves them inside the body to be removed another day and sometimes, as in the case of a man with a brain tumour, she stuffs it in one ear and pulls it, streaked with blood, out of the other. The cotton wool is believed to 'suck up' the disease.

A team of Swiss scientists once came to scrutinize this procedure. They provided Josephine with some cotton wool which they had previously treated with radioactive cobalt. She did her disappearing act into the abdomen of a patient, and sure enough, by using a geiger counter, the scientists were able to locate the exact position of the cotton wool in the body.

The sheer quantities of matter and the incredibly fast turnover, coupled with the fact that at all times I was closely observing her hands and could see everything that was going on, seemed to rule out sleight-of-hand. Financial gain is unlikely to be a motive. Most patients leave just a peso or two in the box. Once again, I never saw the skin actually part, but from Josephine's empty, clean hands all this stuff would appear. If there were concealed capsules or phials there would need to have been a great number of them and very elaborate preparations would have been required. I am truly puzzled. Magic is obviously a very important part of the process here and the whole 'seeing is believing' aspect contributes enormously to the cure, and yet there seems to be something more than a skilful hoax going on. I would be prepared to state categorically that the patient's body is not actually opened although I have seen some remarkably convincing photographs and there are people who would shout me down. Many scientists and psychic researchers are convinced that stuff is materializing from inside the body. Some have offered the explanation that the incisions are happening in the astral body and by some trick of perception the harmful lumps can be expelled without piercing the skin. But the majority have pronounced it all fraud and trickery.

I think the whole argument about whether it does or doesn't 'happen', in the accepted sense of the word, is off beam. It happens on some level, and to be forever trying to discredit it or catch the healers out seems an inappropriate response, as well as damaging to the atmosphere of hope and trust which is activating the patients' own immune systems.

Too much importance is attached to the operation, and focusing on the fake or genuine controversy results in the whole procedure's not being seen in its entirety. I think we are in the realm of symbols, metaphors and visualizations again – another reality from another dimension of the mind's extraordinary capacity for make-believe.

There was certainly nothing very spiritual about the atmosphere – just a great crush of patients and their relatives milling about. Personally I wasn't drawn to the conveyor-belt high-turnover format. It was as impersonal and perfunctory as an English outpatients' clinic in a busy hospital and lacked that quality of unconditional positive regard and individual attention that I saw Placido give – but Josephine's popularity must reflect the degree of success she has. Also, for a patient, the prospect of a thrilling drama with you as the star is undeniably attractive. To see the 'proof' – yards of macaroni or handfuls of bloody straw – materialize from your abdomen and to hear the gasps of astonishment from the spectators, must be very satisfying and exonerating – a public witnessing of the severity of your affliction. 'No wonder I felt ill!' Its subsequent banishment would then allow you to put it decently behind you and let go.

The figure usually quoted as a success rate for the Filipino faith healers is thirty per cent, which is pretty impressive when you consider that most patients who come here have already been written off by orthodox medicine.

Rae allowed me to photograph her treatment. Josephine immediately diagnosed her problem as being caused by a combination of spinal misalignment, brain damage (from a car accident) and an over-active thyroid gland. She had a comparatively lengthy treatment, involving stripping off behind the flimsy curtain, wads of cotton wool being magicked into her eye sockets and out again, and some white pus-like fluid extracted from her throat – lots of blood and gore. The whole thing didn't take more than five minutes.

Melvin had a gruesome eyeball session where Josephine told him to relax more, then appeared to pop one eye out of the socket, remove several fibrous clots and a caterpillar and replace it! He looked as if he was going to be sick but had to acknowledge that he felt no pain. After three hours and some hundred operations I decided to push off. The atmosphere wasn't really conducive to learning and Josephine was too busy to talk or answer questions. The place looked like a slaughterhouse and was terribly hot.

Rae and Melvin wanted to stay a bit longer – Rae's great bulk standing on a bench to see better, towering above the little Filipinos and assuming a bizarre attitude of prayer; hands clasped, eyes half-closed, whole body shaking. I don't know if, when she gets the divine palsy, it's an involuntary tic, an exhibitionistic attention-getter, a cosmic orgasm, or a deeply felt entrance of spiritual energy, but it's quite embarrassing to stand next to her!

Anyway, I left them there and got a ride back to the Carmen crossroads where I didn't have to wait long before I could flag down a bus going back to Baguio and jump aboard. Lots of people had cautioned me against travelling alone but if I had listened to all the alarmist scare stories I would never have got anywhere; the market is full of thieves, every other taxi driver is a bandit and it's certainly not safe to take a walk in the countryside. Actually the NPA kidnapping stories I do take seriously, because hot-headed young revolutionaries are so trigger-happy, but beyond taking reasonable precautions and not asking for trouble, everyone I met was kind and helpful.

When I arrived for my appointment with Placido, he told me that the Central American guy I'd watched him treat the other day hadn't bothered to come back for his second appointment. Placido had sat and waited for him – one of the obvious hazards of not charging anything. He was philosophical but plainly hurt. I got the feeling he had suffered some snubs and knocks in his time. A lot of foreign patients treat the healers like a row of fruit machines, running from one to another, trying their luck, seeking a miracle, hoping to hit the jackpot and go home with their pockets full of unearned health.

I had hoped Placido would have a few more patients today but apparently the explosive political situation has scared off many overseas visitors. We talked some more instead. How can it be, I asked, that matter can be removed from the body without leaving any visible mark? 'I don't know,' he answered, shrugging

his shoulders, 'but to me, it feels just as if I were dipping m
fingers into a glass of water. The molecules part effortlessly an
come together again leaving no trace when I withdraw them.'

One of the little books I bought here, *The Truth Behind Fait
Healing in the Philippines* by Jaime Licauco, offers this attemp
at a rational explanation:

'. . . What happens during a healing session involving psych
surgery goes beyond physical science and beyond the physica
senses of man. Unless we change our fundamental assumptior
regarding the nature of the physical universe and admit th
existence of other levels of reality within which our healers ac
then no explanation is possible or believable.' He says that rathe
than call it 'surgery', which is misleading, we should regard it a
'interpenetration into the different levels or dimensions of man
being and as materialising the diseased tissues into the visib
dimension . . . I believe that the healers are able, through intens
concentration, to form a strong etheric force or energy aroun
their hands, specially at the finger-tips which can part and pene
trate matter at the cellular or even sub-atomic levels where matte
and energy are interchangeable.'

Placido showed me a lot of photos of himself at work and
load of testimonies from grateful ex-patients including Ton
Roche, the tennis star, doubles partner of John Newcombe, wh
was cured of painful tennis elbow that nearly ended his career . .
A Swiss woman who suffered from arthritis of the spine had t
be carried on and off the plane to get here. She was completel
healed and has since written a book about her experience, *Le
Doigts de Dieu*. An Australian man with malignant tumours i
his foot decided to try faith healing as one last desperate attemp
to rid his body of the cancer before having his foot amputated
Placido cured him. A professional dancer who had both hee
smashed in a rock-climbing accident is now renewed and dancin
again. A little boy born with a limb deformity can now walk
The father of a child with muscular dystrophy sent a photo an
wrote, 'Jimmy and I are now hill climbing together for the fir
time in six years.'

The Australian *Sunday Mirror* and Philippine Airways onc

flew a group of thirty-eight readers out to see him. One woman with a paralysed jaw had been living on a liquid diet for years. She was so bombed out on painkillers that her life expectancy was only six months. There was a photo of her taking a big bite out of an apple for the first time in five years.

'What makes a good healer?' I asked Placido. He thought for a while then said, 'I think it is a sacred desire which then unleashes a powerful energy. There is only one source and that is the great creator of the universe – doesn't matter what you call it – to me that is God, but it is still there even if a person claims not to be religious.' He also said that as he understood it, the purpose of healing was change. 'A person must reform in order to change their negativity to positivity. Not everyone gets better.' (That word 're-form' again.)

He told me the story of a Dutchman with a brain tumour who came to see him. He was nearly a hopeless case but Placido treated him and within five months he could walk again. As he got better he returned to his bad old ways and within a year he had crashed himself up in a sports car. He paid for Placido to fly over and treat him again but he died in hospital. Placido was vilified in the press as a quack and even accused of black magic, but, as he says, 'I stand with my pure heart. I did my best but I cannot cure death. That was his destiny. The man did not want to change.'

'Why are people so anxious to discredit faith healers?' I asked. 'Because they are trained to believe that their knowledge is the only one. Medical science is very arrogant. There are many different forms of perception. All human beings are subject to limitations and they do not know everything, but I will never be ashamed to defend the art of healing.' I asked him, in view of what I'd seen at Josephine's, what his views were on witchcraft. He said that a negative mind can attract negative forces, and in such cases he would define the resulting illness as possession by evil spirits, to be countered by magic.

Placido also had some sad stories. A dying boy in a coma was brought to him by his father. His breathing was obstructed and his heartbeat faint. Placido felt this was a case for modern medicine so he sent him quickly to the hospital. But because the man was poor and dirty they didn't let him in and the child died. (It's important to remember that many of the poor patients who come to the healers have had bad experiences of this nature – dismissive or heartless treatment.)

Had his powers ever deserted him? I asked. 'Sometimes I am hard-headed, then I get abandoned,' he answered, 'but nearly always when I go into my deep concentration I can switch on my clairvoyance and the energy starts to flow through me. There is a time to every purpose. The rest of the time I am a normal man.'

He offered to help me increase my own healing skills by 'opening up my third eye and stimulating my pineal gland'. A less trustful person might have suspected the emergence of 'normal man' at this point – but it actually never occurred to me. I was very curious to experience a treatment and was always rather sorry I had nothing dramatic which needed curing.

I lay on the table, and with Kenny, his assistant, in attendance as mopper-up, Placido put his hand over my forehead and made an invocation in Tagalog. He held my ankles, knees, wrists and elbows in turn (very similar to Rosalyn Bruyere's 'chelation' technique), then suddenly dived into my forehead with a wrenching sound. It didn't exactly hurt but felt rather uncomfortable, as if the skin were being pressed hard with the bristles of a hairbrush – hard enough to have left a mark or scratch. Something wet trickled down the side of my face. He then closed up the 'opening' and gently massaged my head, face and neck. Finally he gave me a general energy balancing.

His hands were powerful and gave off a lot of heat. They were also calming and reassuring, kindly but impersonal. It was a very sincere and genuine gift for which I am touched and grateful. The hallmark of all the good healers I have met is a willingness to be generous. Sharing and disseminating their knowledge and skills, they have no need to cultivate their own charisma or jealously to guard their power for themselves.

'Your capacity will be increased,' said Placido, 'and you can now double the number of patients you help.' I looked in the mirror. Not a sign of anything except a bit of blood on my collar. I can't say I felt any startling enlightenment but I was happy to be joined in some way to the loving web of good work that is accomplished here.

Since his own practice is so quiet at the moment, he asked if I would like to meet his old friend Lawrence Cacteng, another healer working in much the same way, but using more herbal remedies. He and Lawrence are from the same village in the north of Luzon Island and have known each other all their lives. Kenny walked me over to his house.

Lawrence is a short, delicate man with classical Bontoc Indian features and a shock of hair brushed forward – very sweet-looking with an enchanting smile and modest manner. I liked him straight away.

A patient arrived almost immediately – a young, nervous Filipino woman suffering from terrible abdominal cramps and menstrual problems. Her face was quite grey from continual pain. This was her fourth visit and I asked if I could help. She winced and tensed as soon as Lawrence started to work on her so I just gently held her hand and head for moral support until the treatment was finished. She relaxed a lot and Lawrence said my presence made a difference, I was useful to have around, so I stayed and assisted him all day. He never tried to conceal anything he was doing and I had a pretty clear view at all times. Like the other healers he operated with amazing speed but always what impressed me more than the bloody part was the infinite tenderness and concentration with which he treated each patient, listening, talking in his unhurried, unruffled way, massaging with his special coconut oil containing cayenne pepper, vinegar and myrrh (Jack Schwartz had a high regard for cayenne pepper too).

Like Placido, he puts his best efforts into this part: soothing, calming, balancing and channelling energy. He told the young woman that she wouldn't need any further treatments, and she left smiling, saying the pain had gone.

Next, a very fat New Zealand woman came in. She was suffering from extensive bruising and a jarred spine following a nasty fall on her tail bone. She had been over to the Philippines for treatment on two or three previous occasions and it occurred to me as I watched the caring way Lawrence and his assistant ministered to her bloated, unattractive body that the tender attentions and devoted focus of the kindly hands of two men touching and stroking her were not an inconsiderable part of the healing process for a lonely middle-aged woman. I'm sure that touch deprivation constitutes as serious a threat to health and well-being as dietary deficiencies.

We all held her and it was fascinating to observe the actual physiological changes which took place: her voice became slower and quieter; her breathing rate deepened; her whole body became calm and relaxed. Lawrence removed some clotted lumps from her leg and almost immediately the blue-black ugly, bruised skin turned pink. I placed my hand on her lower back while she was in this very receptive state and tried to visualize a wash of green-coloured light dissipating the inflammation, reducing the swelling and removing the pain. She cried a bit as some old buried grief welled up in her, and I thought of Elisabeth Kübler-Ross and the marvellous work she does in helping people with their 'unfinished business', their old heavy baggage.

This wasn't the time or the place to do that kind of work but I think the process had begun for her and I told her about the Life, Death and Transition workshops so that she could follow it up if ever the opportunity presented itself. I'm so excited by this global jigsaw. All the pieces have a place in the whole picture.

Lawrence comes, he told me, from a family of healers and herbalists – his mother used to cure people by the old shamanic technique of sucking the disease out of them and spitting it away. He discovered his own gifts as a child, when during a typhoon a tree fell and crushed his companion. All alone and with no alternative, he instinctively applied magnetic healing, then carried the boy on his back home to their remote mountain village. The broken leg swelled painfully but Lawrence continued to do the healing and massage for a week and the leg healed well.

'I have always had a strong faith,' he said. 'In my opinion, healing works because we are all connected to God. I firmly believe that without Him there is no life and healers are powerless.

I have an unshakable faith in that tremendous force – it is the source of hope and of peace. Life is useless without grasping that.'

He resisted healing as a kid because he was more interested in being a kid, but gradually the vocation sneaked up on him. He has a very highly developed sensitivity to what he calls 'the vibrations' and makes his diagnoses according to these clairvoyant observations and clairsentient touchings. He also spends quite a long time with each patient just talking, trying to hear 'if there are any hidden reasons for the sickness'. He believes that most illness arises when there is an emotional, physical and spiritual imbalance. His job, as he sees it, is to restore harmony. 'That's common sense,' he said.

It's a humbling thought that this wisdom we have taken so long to grasp in the West is mere common sense to a man with no medical training and very little education.

I have heard criticisms of the Filipino healers, calling them ignorant and naive. How arrogant! Rational deductions, education and training could be more likely to hamper than to enhance their gifts. It requires great surrender to be the 'instrument' and I believe that genuine humility rather than great intelligence is probably the key prerequisite.

Learning to preserve one's identity, one's individuality, one's ethical integrity, and yet surrender willingly to that which is greater than oneself creates the healing link and generates the healing energy. 'Western people think too much,' said Lawrence, smiling. 'There are some things for which no explanation is possible. But a healer is only human. Too much pressure from Europeans may tempt him to resort to tricks.'

He was scornful of a well-known, wealthy healer here who refused to treat AIDS cases. 'A true healer should never refuse any request,' he said. 'God will protect him.' He claims that the AIDS virus will respond to magnetic healing – the strongest tool in his healing armoury. This is the direct flow of pure energy from the source of life – God, if you like. He uses it in combination with other therapies such as herbal oils and infusions, acupressure, massage, diet and fasting, psychic surgery, water therapy, animal sacrifice, clay packs, and burial up to the neck in volcanic sand on the beach of nearby San Fernando (effective for rheumatism, arthritis and skin complaints) – all depending on what the disease is and what kind of person is manifesting it.

When I asked him what he thought was the most important quality a healer should have, he answered, 'Sincerity. If a person is not sincere there can be no love and compassion.'

Lawrence is a poor man who does not charge for his services. What donations he receives he is putting towards his dream of building a healing clinic with a chapel. He has already purchased a plot of land and the building work has begun. Meanwhile, his wife's earnings as a teacher help keep the family fed, although it means their having to live apart. Her job is one hundred and fifty miles away in their home village.

I liked him so much and would feel no hesitation in recommending someone to come either to him or to Placido for healing. Both are gentle and devout men with a love of humanity and a desire to alleviate suffering. They are very different from the highly commercial and flamboyant exploiters who capitalize on desperation and need. Maybe they too started out with genuine motives but became corrupted by success. I hope that never happens to Placido and Lawrence.

At the end of the day we said goodbye with a lot of affectionate feeling on both sides and a knowledge that we had worked well together. I walked down to the market and bought myself a little selection of things to eat from the street vendors: an ear of roasted corn, a tiny paper cone of sweet-potato chips, a fried banana on a stick, and a couple of passion fruits. What a supper! I felt happy and rather high – head buzzing with everything I'd seen.

I got back to my *pension* to find a message from the Rev. Philip Malicdan, one of the healers I'd tried to contact on my first day. He had just returned from a visit to Stockholm. We spoke on the phone. I told him I had been planning to leave early in the morning for Manila but if he was to be seeing any patients I would be glad to come over to meet him and watch him work before I left. He had two people coming so we made an apppointment to meet at his place.

The Rev. has a much grander establishment than most, and his wife showed me into his lounge where he was waiting to receive me – a dapper slick gentleman with gold teeth, embroidered shirt, navy-blue suit and shiny patent-leather shoes. He is President of the Cultural Minorities Spiritual Fraternization, as proclaimed by a framed certificate on his wall which also states that he is authorized to solemnize marriages.

His story is that he comes from a poor Igorot family from Bontoc Mountain Province where his great-grandparents and his parents were all noted healers. He went to a theological seminary when he left school and is ordained as a Lutheran minister, but healing always seemed to be his vocation. He was the only child in that generation of his family to inherit the gift and used to travel around with his parents from place to place in the mountains, healing people.

The source of the family power is a special cave where the chosen are called for a period of fasting and meditation. He is the sixty-ninth member of the family to participate in this ancient tradition.

His patients today were two poor miners from the gold mines just outside Baguio. They were waiting nervously in the front room. I was invited to watch and photograph the operations. The first man had an ulcer caused by too much drinking, the second had gall bladder problems and pain in his lower back from working bent over underground.

We began by all joining hands in a circle and praying for healing. Both patients received dramatic surgery with remarkable snapping and tearing sounds accompanying the removal of the nasties. I had the clearest possible view of the healer's hands from only a few inches away.

First, he wipes the area clean. With the tips of his rigid fingers he traces around its edge, then begins to rub up and down with his forefingers crossing one another. He appears to mark out a small triangle, then, with his eyes closed and an expression of intense concentration, he stabs his fingers into the flesh and wrenches out the lumps and clots while the blood wells up.

He had on an immaculate white and silky long-sleeved polyester shirt and not so much as a drop of blood appeared on his cuffs. Following the 'surgery', he gives a gentle massage with pure coconut oil containing the crushed sun-dried vine root, llastico, which has first been boiled in oil and then strained (he gave me a jar of this to take home).

He told me that during the operations he concentrates so intensely that he begins to visualize the body as becoming semi-fluid and therefore easy to penetrate.

I simply cannot explain what happens. Everything I know about the human body tells me that you cannot open up the intricate layers of skin, tissue and muscle to wrench out lumps of matter from inside, causing no pain and leaving no wound. But then the seemingly impossible is also achieved by Fijian fire-walkers who walk across beds of red-hot coals without burning their feet; by karate experts who chop concrete blocks in half with their bare hands, and by chaps like Jack Schwartz, who stick knitting needles through their cheeks and draw them out again leaving no scar and no bleeding.

In spite of everything I've seen here my rational mind still comes down on the side of a brilliant sleight-of-hand and yet the treatment rooms are so bare and simple, the equipment so basic, the amount of blood and guts so plentiful that I don't know how they could keep up the conspiracy of deception for so long. If it was a clever con trick surely some mole would have blown the method by now. Even if it meant killing the goose that laid the golden egg, there are enough greedy individuals around who would have compromised the system for personal gain. Anyhow, no foreign scientist or observer seems yet to have given a convincing explanation. Concealed razor blades; slivers of mica; condoms filled with blood; a chemical that turns red when mixed with water – none of these could possibly be the answer. So I am content, for the time being, to let the puzzle remain unsolved.

When the two men had gone, Philip offered to give me a lift all the way to Manila where he had some business. I asked him, on the journey, why such great healing activity has sprung up here and nowhere else in the world. He said that there seems to be something about the geographical location of the Philippines;

the energy comes up from the ground. That may sound a bit far-fetched but, after all, earth energy and ley-lines were just what Bruce MacManaway talked about.

I think Philip is a good healer and he produced lots of testimonies, photos and stories about his successful cases, including a touching letter from a fifteen-year-old girl in Australia, thanking him for having healed her father of lung cancer; a newspaper report about a man with rare cancer of the chest cavity now leading a normal life; and a photo of a bonny new baby sent by a woman who had previously been unable to conceive. But I think he is at that crucial transitionary stage which many healers don't seem to have survived unsullied. Nobody gets rich tending poor peasants and miners for a couple of pesos a time. The scent of possible international recognition and a more prosperous lifestyle for this ordinary man with a wife and seven kids may make the temptation of commercial shenanigans almost too great to resist. I can understand, too, how the bitter rivalries and petty jealousies arise. The Republic of the Philippines is a poor one and the chance for a leg-up into the world of smart hotels, glamour and fame makes people greedy and scheming.

All the way down the mountain road in the car, Philip spent a lot of time hustling me about trying to arrange groups of English patients to come to the Philippines or clubbing together to bring him over to England. The irony is that the very qualities of simple faith and sincerity that make the Filipino healers so remarkable are often the first casualties of foreign patronage. Nobody seems immune.

Even Rustico Villamor is not immune – the healer whose little shack I visited on the first day only to learn from his wife that he was away in Austria. Philip told me that the reason he spends so much time in Austria is that he has married an Austrian woman in order to enjoy the benefits of European citizenship. He stays several months a year abroad and his poor wife back here endures the compromise stoically as long as the earnings keep coming in.

Philip was also once tempted to marry a willing Austrian lady, he told me, but then thought better of it, preferring to wait until an English one happened along! He flashed his gold teeth at me seductively. He is very envious of the status accorded British or American passport-holders. I pointed out that Christians are only supposed to be allowed one wife. 'That's a problem,' he agreed. But I think quite a few arrangements to get round this have been countenanced in order to obtain the precious foothold of citizenship in a land of more opportunity.

He kept hinting at ways we might do partnership deals together and the very artlessness of his scheming was both sad and poignant. I would hate to give the impression that this in any way makes him less effective as a healer. Many people all over the world would testify to his skills, and he already travels widely, sponsored by grateful ex-patients, but I fear he could be in danger of becoming like Jun Labo if he's not careful. I heard, for instance, from one Swiss patient, that Tony Agpaoa, the most famous Filipino healer of them all, who died three years ago at the height of his fame from a massive cerebral haemorrhage, used to ask $1,000 for a healing in advance! Also that towards the end of his short life, the greater his popularity became, the less he was able to achieve. The more money he made, the more frequently his powers deserted him. Commercial success does not seem to be compatible with the basic principles of healing.

As we neared Manila, the Rev. made his last bid. He noticed that my ankles were swollen from all the walking and altitude changes. Perhaps if I cared to come to his hotel that evening he could give me some healing and I, in turn, could heal his hypertension! I made my excuses and asked the driver to drop me off at my borrowed flat, where my new friends downstairs welcomed me in and cooked me a wonderful supper of fried fish and vegetables in coconut milk. A letter was waiting for me from home and I had my first proper shower and hair wash for a week. Bliss!

My friends offered to give me an insider's unorthodox, non-tourist tour of the city on my last day. After this glimpse of the unimaginable poverty and hardship of which most people's lives here consist, I could understand much better the pressures on the poor healers to try and improve their lot. The yawning abyss is just waiting there for anyone to tumble into. People scratch a meagre existence selling single cigarettes to passing motorists for a few centavos; or an ounce of peanuts, or a religious calendar. Everyone is trying to sell you something so they can eat today. I saw a tiny naked sleeping baby lying all alone right on the bare concrete pavement with a plastic begging cup beside her.

After wandering through the steaming, teeming streets, where I would not have gone alone, we ended up at a large poor people's church in the middle of Sunday worship – it was a medieval tableau of limbless beggars, incense sellers, and magic-talisman purveyors. Ragged children were sleeping in the alcoves, people were queueing to file round a lurid life-size waxwork effigy of the dead Christ encased in a glass casket with only His feet sticking out, which everyone kissed. Outside were hundreds of little stalls selling herbal medicines, love potions, charms, religious pictures and plastic flowers. Healers, fortune tellers, and astrologers sat on stools curing headaches and reading palms. I bought a couple of bottles of garish medicine and two lumps of magic incense 'to drive away evil spirits'. The faith healers of the Philippines arise out of this rich hue of tribal animistic tradition overlaid with simple fervent Christianity.

In their healing practices they seem to have clung on to a much earlier intuition about the interconnectedness of body, mind and spirit which flourishes still in an atmosphere where miracles are seen as compatible with the laws of nature. Sadly, our dollars and our scepticism seem to have contributed unwittingly to the destruction of this harmonious world view.

I'm glad I saw all this, but it was pretty overwhelming and I flew home that night with a full heart. I loved my time in the Philippines and what I witnessed made me certain that some fine healers are working there. It also convinced me once and for all that true healing comes from within the patient and that a healer's role is to act as a catalyst for change. He or she is the person who helps us to push out the boundaries of the possible and 're-form'. Between them, the healer and the patient create a sacred space and a channel to that abstract concept called the life force.

Anyone coming to the Philippines to seek healing, however, would be well advised to see only those healers who have been personally recommended to them. There is a lot of racketeering going on and I, myself, would stay away from a package deal connected with a travel agency, because I don't like the idea of middlemen profiting from someone else's misfortune and also because I think the adventure, the effort and the pilgrimage are part of the journey towards transformation.

Once having made the decision to try something extraordinary and having chosen a particular healer, I think a patient should then try to be as relaxed and open as possible, investing the venture with hope and optimism, recognizing that healing is not a passive process wherein something is done to one, but involves active participation – a conspiracy of emotional consent – and a commitment to change whatever the outcome.

I told my son about the meeting with Paz Navalta and he was intrigued. While I was away in the Philippines he had come to the decision that it was time to do something about the stalemate in his life. He had already made a decision to stop smoking dope and liked the idea of performing the little orange-juice exorcism to celebrate the occasion and 'discharge the low forces' weighing him down.

I squeezed three fresh oranges and said the magic words, then we lit a candle and he solemnly drank the potion. It sounds silly but it was actually a very beautiful little ceremony. I held him in my arms – awkward, bolshie, street-wise, heartbreaking, six-foot-three-inches baby boy that I love so much.

Two weeks later he grew up, married his beautiful girlfriend – and they lived happily ever after, I hope.

The story of this quest really started with him, but the lessons I learned along the way are that all healing is self-healing and that each person's journey is his or her own. There is no one particular starting point and wherever you choose to dip your toe into the water the ripples will spread, leading your vision further and further out, with no limits other than your own willingness to see. Inner blindness seems to me to be a source of much disease (dis-ease). So much of what we do is unconscious. We trudge, unquestioning, in well-worn tramlines like blinkered mules in a coal mine.

Healing is a journey into the inner world to discover who we are and why we do the things we do. It is a commitment to trying to understand the relationship between mind and body and what we use illness *for*. It is an attempt, finally, to free ourselves from the chains of habit. Most people assume they don't know enough about their own bodies to understand what's going on but I've learned that we know a lot more than we think. Many levels of knowing are available to us if only we dare to open ourselves to the possibilities.

The trouble for the novice seeker is the confusing multiplicity of paths that exist to choose from. There are hundreds of therapies on the market. None of them has all the answers, all of them have some of the answers. It doesn't really matter where you start. One of the big dangers of exploration in this field is that everyone tells you their way is *the* way. The vital thing is to retain a sense of humour and to listen to your heart – you will eventually discover what is right for you. 'The real voyage of discovery consists not in seeking new lands but in seeing with new eyes,' said Proust.

Healing is a miraculous phenomenon and one of mankind's greatest gifts. To me, the one continuous thread that wove together all the good healers I met was their capacity for unconditional love. I think therein lies the magic. It brings with it the gift of wings and the freedom to soar to a place where anything is possible. So much illness arises as a defence against life – a coping strategy. Gradually dismantling the defences means allowing the life force to flow in. Health is more than just an absence of disease, it is an embracing of life.

SOME FURTHER READING

CHAPTER 1

C. G. Jung, *Man and His Symbols*, Picador, 1978
Gallegos and Rennick, *Inner Journeys: Visualization in Growth and Therapy*, Turnstone Press, 1984
Idries Shah, *Tales of the Dervishes*, Octagon Press, 1982
Idries Shah, *The Way of the Sufi*, Penguin, 1974
Don Copeland, *So You Want to Be a Healer*, National Federation of Spiritual Healers, 1981
Lorna Horstmann, *A Handbook of Healing*, National Federation of Spiritual Healers, 1962
Michal J. Eastcott, *The Silent Path*, Rider & Co, 1983
Virginia Hanson, *Approaches to Meditation*, Quest Books (Illinois), 1973
Richard Gordon, *Your Healing Hands*, Unity Press (California), 1978
W. Brugh Joy, *Joy's Way*, J. P. Tarcher (Los Angeles), 1979

CHAPTER 2

Elisabeth Kübler-Ross and Mal Warshaw, *Working It Through*, Macmillan (New York), 1982

CHAPTER 3

Bruce MacManaway with Johanna Turcan, *Healing*, Thorsons, 1983

Diane Mariechild, *Mother Wit*, The Crossing Press (USA), 1981, distributed in the UK by Airlift Book Co., London
Albright and Albright (ed.), *Mind, Body and Spirit*, Thule Press (now The Findhorn Press), 1981
Francis Hitching, *Earth Magic*, Cassell, 1976
Colin Wilson, *The Occult*, Panther (now Grafton), 1979
Colin Wilson, *Mysteries*, Panther (now Grafton), 1979
Colin Wilson, *Frankenstein's Castle*, Ashgrove Press, 1980

CHAPTER 4

Lyall Watson, *Gifts of Unknown Things*, Coronet, 1977
Lyall Watson, *The Lightning Bird*, Coronet, 1983
Sudhir Kakar, *Shamans, Mystics and Doctors*, Unwin, 1984

CHAPTER 5

George Trevelyan, *A Vision of the Aquarian Age*, Coventure Ltd, 1977
Lynn Andrews, *Medicine Woman*, Routledge & Kegan Paul, 1984

CHAPTER 6

Namkhai Norbu, *The Mirror: Advice on Presence and Awareness*, Shang-Shung Editions (Arcidosso Grosetto, Italy), 1983
Sheldon B. Kopp, *If You Meet the Buddha on the Road, Kill Him!*, Sheldon Press, 1974

CHAPTER 7

Jack Schwartz, *Human Energy Systems*, Dutton (New York), 1980
C. G. Jung, *Memories, Dreams, Reflections*, Flamingo, 1983
Nona Coxhead and Maxwell Cade, *The Awakened Mind*, Wildwood House, 1980
Annie Wilson and Lilla Bel:, *What Colour Are You?*, Turnstone Press, 1981

CHAPTER 8

Ian Gawler, *You Can Conquer Cancer*, Thorsons, 1986
Jennifer Isaacs, *Australian Dreaming: 40,000 Years of Aboriginal History*, Lansdowne Press (Sydney), 1980
Bill Neidjie, *Kakadu Man*, Mybrood P/L Ltd (New South Wales), 1985
Alan Moorehead, *The Fatal Impact*, Penguin, 1968

CHAPTER 9

Janice Reid, *Sorcerors and Healing Spirits*, Australian National University Press (Sydney), 1983
Mary Chamberlain, *Old Wives' Tales*, Virago, 1981
J. M. Cohen and J. F. Phipps, *The Common Experience*, Rider: Element Books, 1979
Joseph Head and S. L. Cranston, *Reincarnation*, Quest Books (Illinois), 1975

CHAPTER 10

Jaime Licauco, *The Magicians of God*, National Book Store, Manila (Philippines), 1981
Harold Sherman, *Wonder Healers of the Philippines*, DeVorss (Los Angeles), 1967
George W. Meek, *Healers and the Healing Process*, Quest Books (Illinois), 1977
Gert Chesi, *Faith Healers in the Philippines*, Morgan (New York), 1981
Jaime Licauco, *The Truth Behind Faith Healing in the Philippines*, National Book Store, Manila (Philippines), 1981

and additionally:

Richard Grossinger, *Planet Medicine*, Shambhala Publications (Boston), 1982
Brian Inglis, *Fringe Medicine*, Faber & Faber, 1964

Brian Inglis and Ruth West, *The Alternative Health Guide*,
   Mermaid Books, 1984
Gaston St Pierre and Debbie Boater, *Metamorphic Technique*,
   Element Books, 1982
Khalil Gibran, *The Prophet*, Pan, 1980
Piero Ferrucci, *What We May Be*, Turnstone Press, 1982
David Harvey, *The Power to Heal*, Aquarian Press, 1983

NOTE: Wherever they are not in the UK, publishers are located by
   place names in brackets.

USEFUL ADDRESSES

Aletheia HEART Center
1809 N.99 Highway
Ashland
Oregon 97520
United States of America

Amethyst
Annacrivey Wood
Enniskerry
Co Wicklow
Eire

Churches Council for Health
    and Healing
Marylebone Road
London NW1 5LT

The Elisabeth Kübler-Ross
    Center
South Rt 616
Head Waters
Virginia 24442
United States of America

   (U.K.) Shanti Nilaya
   PO Box 212
   London NW8 7NW

Healing Light Center
204 E Wilson
Glendale
California 91206
United States of America

Human Potential Resources
(a quarterly directory)
LFG Ltd
HP12
Subscription Department
PO Box 10
Lincoln LN5 8XE

Institute of Complementary
    Medicine
21 Portland Place
London W1N 3AF

Metamorphic Association
67 Ritherdon Road
London SW1 8QE

National Federation of
  Spiritual Healers
Old Manor Farm Studio
Church Street
Sunbury-on-Thames
Middx. TW16 6RG

Westbank Healing and
  Teaching Centre
Strathmiglo
Fife
Scotland KY14 7QP

The Wrekin Trust
Marbury House
St Owen Street
Hereford